T0080284

BIRTH CONTROL

WHAT EVERYONE NEEDS TO KNOW®

BIRTH CONTROL
WHAT EVERYONE NEEDS TO KNOW®

BETH SUNDSTROM AND CARA DELAY

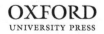

OXFORD
UNIVERSITY PRESS

OXFORD
UNIVERSITY PRESS

Oxford University Press is a department of the University of Oxford. It furthers the University's objective of excellence in research, scholarship, and education by publishing worldwide. Oxford is a registered trade mark of Oxford University Press in the UK and certain other countries.

"What Everyone Needs to Know" is a registered trademark of Oxford University Press

Published in the United States of America by Oxford University Press 198 Madison Avenue, New York, NY 10016, United States of America.

© Oxford University Press 2020

All rights reserved. No part of this publication may be reproduced, stored in a retrieval system, or transmitted, in any form or by any means, without the prior permission in writing of Oxford University Press, or as expressly permitted by law, by license, or under terms agreed with the appropriate reproduction rights organization. Inquiries concerning reproduction outside the scope of the above should be sent to the Rights Department, Oxford University Press, at the address above.

You must not circulate this work in any other form and you must impose this same condition on any acquirer.

Library of Congress Cataloging-in-Publication Data
Names: Sundstrom, Beth, 1983– author. | Delay, Cara, 1971– author.
Title: Birth control : what everyone needs to know® /
Beth Sundstrom and Cara Delay.
Description: New York, NY : Oxford University Press, 2020. |
Series: What everyone needs to know® |
Includes bibliographical references and index.
Identifiers: LCCN 2019048256 (print) | LCCN 2019048257 (ebook) |
ISBN 9780190069667 (paperback) | ISBN 9780190069674 (hardback) |
ISBN 9780190069698 (epub)
Subjects: LCSH: Reproductive rights—United States. |
Birth control—United States.
Classification: LCC HQ766.5.U5 S87 2020 (print) |
LCC HQ766.5.U5 (ebook) | DDC 363.9/60973—dc23
LC record available at https://lccn.loc.gov/2019048256
LC ebook record available at https://lccn.loc.gov/2019048257

The resources in this book are intended for use only as a tool to assist clinicians/school-based professionals and should not be used to replace clinical judgment or school-based policies and procedures. The information in this book is not provided as legal advice and/or professional advice on specific situations. While we have attempted to ensure the accuracy of information contained herein, we do not warrant that it is complete or accurate, and we are not legally responsible for errors or omissions.

1 3 5 7 9 8 6 4 2

Paperback printed by LSC Communications, United States of America
Hardbback printed by Bridgeport National Bindery, Inc., United States of America

For Millie and Byrdie—and a generation growing up to expect bodily autonomy and unfettered access to science and technology without fear or judgment

CONTENTS

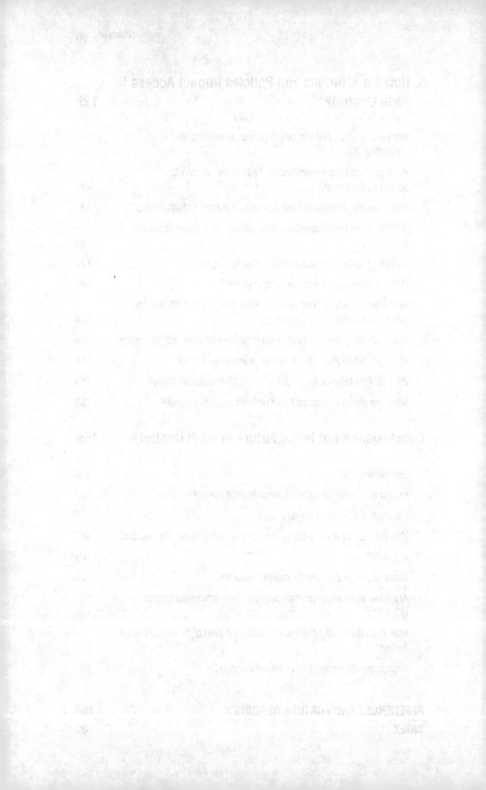

ACKNOWLEDGMENTS

Writing this book has been a labor of love and a collective effort in so many ways. First and foremost, we would like to thank our colleagues at the College of Charleston for their support. The School of Humanities and Social Sciences, the Women's and Gender Studies program, and, especially, the Women's Health Research Team (WHRT) have provided inspiration and encouragement throughout this process. Directing and mentoring faculty and students on the WHRT has provided a source of tireless enthusiasm for this work. We are most thankful for our collaborations with WHRT members, past and present, and particularly Nicole Russo, who helped us prepare this manuscript.

We are indebted to our community of scholars, women's health activists, and organizational partners in the United States and abroad who make our research not only possible but also rewarding. We thank our colleagues at the Medical University of South Carolina (MUSC), the University of South Carolina, Clemson University, Brown University, the Women's Rights and Empowerment Network (WREN), the South Carolina Coalition for Healthy Families, Power to Decide, and Ibis Reproductive Health, among others, for partnering with us and collaborating in this essential research on birth control. We are grateful for our Fulbright U.S. Scholar Research Grant Awards in Ireland for those transformative experiences and for the communities we were fortunate to join at University College Dublin and University College Cork.

The editorial team at Oxford University Press has been a joy to work with. Chad Zimmerman and Chloe Layman in particular have been supportive and enthusiastic at every step of this process. Working with you is an experience that we hope to repeat.

As we struggled to choose a cover image for this book, we were fortunate that Chad Zimmerman came across the amazing feminist artist Ali Harrison. We can think of no better image than Ali's papercut uterus to adorn our book. Thank you, Ali.

We owe the success of our research to the women who participated in our interviews over nearly a decade. We are grateful for your generosity in sharing your time, experiences, and voices. Your stories and voices, which we hope we have done justice to here, are invaluable and need to be heard.

To our friends and families, especially Paris, Bryan, Millie, and Byrdie, we offer our thanks for their patience, encouragement, and generosity of spirit. Thank you for the time and space to write and thank you for listening.

INTRODUCTION

BIRTH CONTROL IN THE UNITED STATES

Birth control is a timely topic. As we finish this book in 2019, contraception and family planning dominate news headlines across the United States. Legal challenges to the 2010 Affordable Care Act's contraceptive mandate continue; the Trump administration has revised decades-old Title X funding policies for contraceptive providers, and both Democratic and Republican legislators recently have come out in support of oral contraceptives over the counter. Meanwhile, a larger discussion of reproductive rights and women's bodily autonomy continues to divide Americans, increasingly on partisan lines. The time is right, then, for a new examination of birth control.

Healthy People 2020 offers national benchmarks to improve the health of women, infants, and families. By 2020, its family planning objectives aim to increase intended pregnancies to 56%, improve access and use of highly effective contraception, and increase birth spacing to 18 months. In this book we provide basic, scientific, and factual information about birth control that can be useful to all people. *Birth Control: What Everyone Needs to Know* is different from other books on birth control, however, in several noteworthy ways. First, it privileges the voices and experiences of ordinary women. Second, it offers a diverse, intersectional perspective grounded in reproductive justice. Third, it draws on our interdisciplinary expertise, placing current issues in a rich historical and cultural context.

Women's voices: Understanding lived experiences

Although reproduction and birth control are experienced primarily by women, accurate information that privileges women's experiences is still rare. Too often, academic researchers and medical practitioners create a divide between objective, fact-based, scientific knowledge and women's personal or subjective experiences. This split, however, can result in a lack of communication between women and "experts" and can even alienate women from essential information. Furthermore, neglecting personal narratives also perpetuates systems of power that continue to privilege the voices of a select few and devalue the essential experiences of ordinary women. The ways that power exists already in our society—in terms of gender, race, sexuality, and more—can affect what is considered valuable in terms of research, leaving behind those with less access to power.

Women's lives and voices are important. Women's stories matter, and telling those stories matters. In this book, we include women's own words and experiences alongside peer-reviewed and scientific information. Guided by a belief that birth control and health care are fundamentally about ordinary people, we privilege the experiences and perspectives of such people. We incorporate women's voices in this book by drawing on a rich body of interviews that we conducted with hundreds of women across several years (2010–2019). These studies featured semistructured in-depth interviews, which involve preparing a list of questions but provide flexibility to develop a "conversational partnership" and allow new ideas to emerge. All research protocol and procedures were approved by university institutional review boards, and all participants provided informed consent to participate and for their words to be used anonymously in publications, such as this book.

Alongside our previously published research findings, these interviews shaped the content of this book and guided our approach to identifying *what everyone needs to know* about birth control. By analyzing the latest scientific evidence about birth control, we address women's questions, concerns and apprehensions about contraception, as well as the ways birth control empowers women and increases access to educational and professional opportunities. Including these interviews provides the opportunity to link medical discourse with women's everyday experiences for the purposes of creating a shared story to improve medical choice and decision making (Sharf & Vanderford, 2008).

The goal of this book is to provide accurate, unbiased scientific information about contraception in the context of women's lived experiences and the realities of how individuals make decisions about birth control. We aim to provide the facts that individuals need to make an informed decision about birth control. There is not one best decision for every person; however, all women and people who can become pregnant deserve access to the best science and evidence without fear or judgment. We encourage individuals to seek the advice of their health-care provider for questions about methods of birth control or family planning. This book is for informational purposes only and is not intended to be a substitute for the professional advice of a health-care provider. We hope that this book will empower women to ask questions and engage in shared decision making with their health-care providers.

In our research, in-depth interviews focused on everything from sex education to contraceptive choice and LGBTQ+ experiences. They allowed individuals to tell their own stories in their own words and therefore validated people's experiences. The results include empowering women within the process of research and encouraging women to be active participants in research. Our interviews served as an opportunity for women to talk about health issues that are important to them, including birth control, and to vocalize their own experiences, needs, wants, and views.

Many women have expressed the realization that they lack a space for sharing their own health experiences. As one woman told us, "gee, I guess I really needed to talk about my health, or something. Thank you. I think I needed this." Our research has empowered participants by providing a protected time and space for women to discuss their own health needs and opinions. In one oral history interview, a woman asked about her views on birth control responded, "Um, nothing negative, you know, just all positive, just giving, giving me the options as a woman, that, you know, giving me the power." While this woman viewed birth control as empowering, she also was empowered by telling her story and having researchers take it seriously.

Intersectionality and reproductive justice

Scholars today who research women and gender employ an intersectional approach. In 1989, lawyer and critical race scholar Kimberlé Crenshaw created the term "intersectionality," sometimes called "intersectional feminism," to describe the magnified oppression that African American women face (Crenshaw, 1989). The Oxford Dictionary defines intersectionality as

> the interconnected nature of social categorizations such as race, class, and gender, regarded as creating overlapping and interdependent systems of discrimination or disadvantage; a theoretical approach based on such a premise.

Intersectionality considers not only gender but also other interlocking categories, including race, ethnicity, class, ability, and sexuality, when analyzing people's status and oppression. It recognizes that people affected by more than one of these categories face compounded levels of oppression. In this book, we apply an intersectional approach. We attempt to move beyond privileging the experiences of middle-class White women only and instead examine how birth control access and usage relates to not only being a woman but also being a person of color, an immigrant, a member of the LGBTQ+ community, a person with a disability, a sex worker, and more.

Intersectional feminism helped inspire a new reproductive justice movement in the 1990s, created by women of color. The World Health Organization and the United Nations describe reproductive rights as human rights. Reproductive justice goes further, however, connecting reproductive rights with social justice and intersectionality (Ross & Solinger, 2017, p. 9). Reproductive justice acknowledges people's rights to decide if and how they become pregnant or stay pregnant and advocates for women's abilities to raise their child(ren) in a safe and healthy environment. First established to recognize and examine the experiences of women of color in the United States, reproductive justice links the social, cultural, environmental, and economic contexts that determine women's physical and mental health (Ross & Solinger, 2017; SisterSong, 2018; Solinger, 2016). Reproductive justice scholars argue that the focus by some feminists on "rights" and "choice" fails to analyze the complicated intersections of sex, race, and class as sources of reproductive oppression and specifically overlooks the experiences of marginalized women (hooks, 1984; Berger & Guidroz, 2010; Roberts, 1997; Ross & Solinger, 2017; SisterSong, 2018). Dorothy Roberts described reproductive justice as a model for human equality and well-being. In her influential book, *Killing the Black Body*, Roberts (1997) argued that the traditional White, middle-class "feminist focus on gender and identification of male domination as the source of reproductive repression often overlooks the importance of racism in shaping our understanding of reproductive liberty and the degree of 'choice' that women really have" (p. 5).

The research that we conducted for this book is grounded firmly in intersectionality and reproductive justice. By moving beyond "rights" rhetoric to diverse lived experiences, we hope to recognize not only how intersectional oppression has decreased people's access to birth control but also how some women have struggled to implement reproductive justice through birth control access and activism. Our goals include "foster[ing] empowerment and emancipation for women and other marginalized groups" as well as "promoting social change and social justice for women" (Sundstrom, 2015, p. 4).

An interdisciplinary and historical perspective

As researchers on a dynamic and interdisciplinary Women's Health Research Team made up of students and professors in Anthropology, Biology, Communication, English, History, Hispanic Studies, and, Public Health, among other disciplines, our approach to birth control disrupts traditional academic boundaries. Our specific training in the fields of Communication, Public Health, Women's Studies, and History means that we bring a unique interdisciplinary focus to this book. In *Birth Control: What Everyone Needs to Know*, we pay particular attention to the history of family planning in the United States and, when relevant, in comparative perspective. We contend that the debates, policies, and issues surrounding birth control that dominate so much of American political, religious, social, and cultural life today cannot be understood without an examination of their origins. For example, recognizing why some Americans today, including immigrants, women of color, and people with disabilities sometimes view contraception as a negative that some providers may force on them requires that we examine the deep historical roots of reproductive coercion and forced sterilization in the United States. The discussions we are having as Americans today about birth control can be enhanced by a careful consideration of not only history but also the media, gender analysis, and public health research.

1

BIRTH CONTROL TODAY

Birth control? Family planning? Contraception? What is the difference?

Talking about family planning, birth control, and contraception can be challenging.

Often confusing, the terminology also has changed over time. Some people even today find it difficult to use clear and direct language relating to birth control. Euphemisms and misnomers abound: condoms are sometimes referred to as "protection," the intrauterine device (IUD) is still known by the outdated "coil," various oral contraceptive pills (OCPs) are widely known as "the pill," emergency contraception is called "the morning after pill," and some refer to female sterilization as "getting your tubes tied."

It is important to discuss correct terminology so that people who can become pregnant and give birth have current, accurate information about birth control. Some terms related to fertility control that may technically have different meanings are often used interchangeably. "Birth control" and "contraception" are the most obvious examples of this. Today, we commonly define birth control as any method intended to prevent or regulate reproduction, including behavioral methods (such as abstinence), fertility awareness methods (including the so-called rhythm method), barrier methods, hormonal methods, and sterilization. Contraception often refers to the use of some-thing artificial, usually a device, hormone, or medication, to prevent pregnancy during or after penile–vaginal sexual intercourse. Birth control thus is a broader, more encompassing term, while contraception is more specific and usually linked to technology and tools or substances, such as the condom, the OCP, and the IUD. Today, however, many people use the terms "birth control" and "contraception" interchangeably to mean the same thing: actions taken by humans to prevent or space pregnancies.

The term "family planning" originally was used as a euphemism for "birth control" in the early twentieth century. It has evolved in recent decades to describe attempts to regulate conception and, often, to space the number of births within a family. Some experts, however, believe that it is less preferable than "contraception" or "birth control" because many who use birth control are not actually attempting to plan families. Others prefer "family planning" because they consider it to be a more inclusive term that may reference couples and includes men, transgender individuals, and gender nonconforming people as well as women. "Family planning" also is more commonly associated with "natural" rather than technological methods and is used in relation to the developing world more frequently than "birth control." The World Health Organization, for example, uses the phrase "family planning/contraception" when discussing birth control globally. According to the United Nations, "family planning" is defined as

> the information, means and methods that allow individuals to decide if and when to have children. This includes a wide range of contraceptives—including pills, implants, intrauterine devices, surgical procedures that limit fertility, and barrier methods such as condoms—as well as non-invasive methods such as the calendar method and abstinence. Family planning also includes

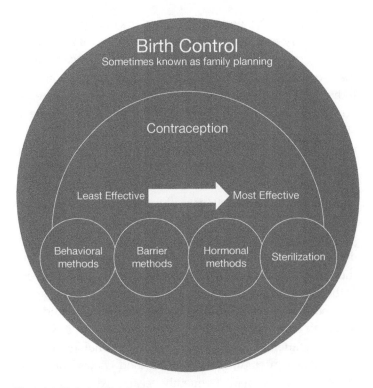

Figure 1.1. Methods of Birth Control.

information about how to become pregnant when it is desirable, as well as treatment of infertility. (United Nations Population Fund, n.d.)

In this book, we use "birth control," "contraception," and "family planning" in accordance with the previous explanations (and as visualized in Figure 1.1).

Is birth control only for women?

No. And here it's important to note that the language associated with gender can also add further confusion to this topic.

People across the gender spectrum, including individuals who identify as transgender, cisgender, nonbinary, or gender nonconforming, may need birth control. *Cisgender* means that you identify as the gender you were assigned at birth. Individuals who identify as transgender, nonbinary, or gender nonconforming may not identify as the gender they were assigned at birth—or with any gender at all. These individuals may or may not choose hormone therapy or surgery as part of their gender journey. All of these factors—along with medical and lifestyle factors to be discussed throughout this book—impact what type of birth control method will be favored by an individual.

While experts increasingly recognize the limits of binary definitions of gender based on biology, terminology surrounding birth control frequently utilizes such concepts. Most of the literature uses the word "woman" to describe those who may become pregnant. In this book, following the guidelines set out in *Reproductive Justice: An Introduction* (Ross & Solinger, 2017), we attempt to employ inclusive terminology and language when discussing birth control and contraception. We use the word "woman" frequently because we are concerned about representing the lived experiences and reproductive decision-making of women, recognizing that eliminating the term "woman" may contribute to the marginalization and oppression of this group. However, we also consciously use "people who can get pregnant and give birth" to recognize that some people who use or need birth control do not identify as women. In this way, we attempt to complicate the gender binary and choose language that recognizes the human right of reproductive autonomy for all persons (Ross & Solinger, 2017, p. 6).

Who needs birth control? Who uses birth control?

Women, men, transgender individuals, and gender nonconforming people need birth control to prevent pregnancy.

Anyone who is sexually active and does not want to become pregnant needs birth control. Some people need birth control to treat a variety of medical conditions, including acne, anemia, heavy menstrual periods, menstrual cramps, polycystic ovary syndrome (PCOS), premenstrual syndrome (PMS), premenstrual dysphoric disorder (PMDD), endometriosis, and primary ovarian insufficiency, among others. Anyone who seeks the net health benefits offered by hormonal contraception needs birth control.

Birth control, however, is still commonly thought of as something for women only. Most studies of birth control focus on women, and most contraceptive methods are designed for women. Today, a vast majority of adolescent and adult American women use some form of birth control. In fact, 99% of women have used contraception at some point in their potential childbearing years. Some women use birth control continuously for decades—as many as 30 years or more—throughout their lifecycle. This means that an average woman will spend more than 75% of her potential reproductive years trying to avoid unwanted or mistimed pregnancies. Studies also suggest a discernible pattern of birth control use across a woman's reproductive lifespan. Many women, for example, begin using condoms at first sexual intercourse, then move on to the pill at a later stage, and then seek sterilization (tubal ligation) after achieving a desired number of children.

While many birth control users are cisgender women or men, people who do not identify in these ways—including transgender or queer individuals and gender nonconforming people—also use birth control. All methods available to cisgender people are also available to transgender people and gender nonconforming individuals. Many LGBTQ+ people engage in sexual behaviors that could result in pregnancy. Importantly, they are also, like cisgender women, in danger of unintended pregnancy via rape or sexual assault: women who identify as non-heterosexual actually have higher rates of unintended pregnancy than do heterosexual women. Still, some people, including many medical professionals, do not fully understand how and why some LGBTQ+ people may need or use birth control. As one interviewee said,

> okay, so I didn't tell my regular doctor, my PCP, that I was gay until this past visit. She was like, "Are you sexually active?" And I was like, "Yeah." And she was like, "Well, are you using condoms, and doing birth control," and all this other stuff, and I was like, "I am sexually active with women so it doesn't really matter that much." And she just said, "Oh, okay." Which wasn't good because you should still be using precautionary measures if you're a woman having sex with women, but, so that was . . . I just don't think she knew how to handle that, because [she was a] small Southern-town doctor.

As we discuss in Chapter 5 of this volume, although most women use birth control, access to it is particularly difficult for some populations. American women who live in rural areas or on federal Indian reservations may have decreased access to pharmacies that supply birth control. Women of color, immigrant and migrant women, including undocumented people, sex workers, and women of a lower socioeconomic position also face obstacles getting contraception.

How likely is it that a woman who does not use a method of birth control will become pregnant?

Intended pregnancies are pregnancies that were planned and desired at the time of conception. Unintended pregnancies, in contrast, are pregnancies that are either unwanted or mistimed. They occur when a woman does not want or intend to become pregnant. In mistimed pregnancies, a woman may want to become pregnant but not necessarily when the pregnancy in question occurs. In unwanted pregnancies, a woman may not want to become pregnant at all in the present or future.

Risk of pregnancy can vary based on several factors, including frequency of penile–vaginal penetrative sex, age, medical conditions, and menstrual cycles. For all people who can become pregnant and give birth, failure to use birth control at all or failure to use it effectively and consistently can result in unintended pregnancy. In fact, those who can become pregnant and give birth and who do not use any method of birth control have an 85% chance of conceiving in the course of a year. In other words, out of 100 women who are not using a method of birth control, 85 will become pregnant in one year. In any given year, across the globe, there are approximately 87 million unplanned pregnancies. However, women who use birth control consistently and correctly account for only 5% of all unintended pregnancies.

What is the current rate of unintended pregnancy in the United States?

In the United States, 50% of all pregnancies are unintended. The United States, in fact, leads the developed world in rates of unintended pregnancies. In 2017, there were 3,855,500 pregnancies in the United States and half of these—1,927,750—were unintended. In 2011, in the United States, 18% of pregnancies were unwanted and 27% of all pregnancies were mistimed. Of unintended pregnancies that occur every year, approximately 40% end in abortion, while 60% result in the birth of an infant.

Beyond these general statistics, there are significant disparities within demographic groups. For example, women below the federal poverty level have markedly higher rates of unplanned pregnancies. For these women, unintended pregnancy levels are more than five times higher than those of women with more economic resources. Younger women and adolescents, particularly aged 15 to 19, also have elevated rates of unintended pregnancies. Women between the ages of

18 and 24, in fact, have the highest levels of unplanned pregnancies. Marital status matters as well: unmarried women are more likely to face unintended pregnancy. In 2017, unmarried women comprised 39.8% of all births in the United States. Almost 70% of pregnancies among young unmarried women aged 20 to 29 are unplanned or unintended. From 2006 to 2012, intended births among women aged 15 to 24 varied by partner status:

- Married women: 60% of births intended
- Cohabiting women: 42% of births intended
- Unmarried non-cohabiting women: 21% of births intended (Mosher, 2012)

Furthermore, educational level has an impact: women without a high school diploma have much higher rates of unintended pregnancy (73 per 1,000) than do women with a high school and/or college-level education. Women with lower levels of completed education have twice as many reported contraceptive failures than women with some level of higher education.

Other demographic factors in unwanted or mistimed conceptions are race and ethnicity. The unintended pregnancy rate for African American and Hispanic women, for example, far exceeds that of White women. Hispanic women have double the levels of unintended pregnancy than do non-Hispanic White women. The reasons for this are complex. First, many women of color often have less access to contraception and health-care services. Furthermore, a history of reproductive violence and coercion against women of color in the United States, which we discuss in more detail in Chapter 2 of this volume, also affects these women's perceptions of birth control, possibly resulting in lower contraceptive use.

Women subject to intimate partner violence are also at an elevated risk of reproductive coercion and unintended pregnancy. Some abusers coerce or force women into sexual activity and/or prevent them from using effective birth control.

Indeed, in some cases, they do so as part of the abuse: to extend further control over their partners. Experience with not only intimate partner violence but also non-voluntary first intercourse is linked to higher rates of mistimed or unwanted pregnancies as well.

Of course, many of the characteristics discussed in this section intersect: poverty often is related to educational status, age, and race or ethnicity. It is important, therefore, to recognize the multiple and overlapping factors that contribute to rates of unintended pregnancy and to design policies and public health strategies that address these intersecting factors.

In the 2010s, new research suggested that rates of unintended pregnancy, particularly among adolescents, were declining in the United States. By 2017, a record low number of American teens reported unintended pregnancies. Although there is no clear consensus on the cause of this decline, most researchers believe that teenage pregnancy rates have slowed because of increased birth control usage and comprehensive sexual health education. Still, unintended pregnancy rates for American women of all age groups remain high compared to those for other developed countries. Birth control offers people the opportunity to prevent pregnancy, plan and space their births, or have no births at all. Yet only half of sexually active American women consistently use birth control.

What are the health effects of unintended pregnancy on women and infants?

Unintended pregnancies often result in poor maternal and child outcomes. Unwanted, rather than mistimed, pregnancies are the most strongly associated with a range of detrimental health effects for women and for infants, but both can have negative effects. One of the most important consequences of unintended pregnancy for people who can become pregnant and give birth is a lack of prenatal care or delayed prenatal care. Women with unintended pregnancies initiate and receive less prenatal care than women with intended pregnancies. People confronting unintended pregnancies generally seek prenatal care later than those whose pregnancies are planned or expected. In addition, risky lifestyle behaviors also may be associated with unintended pregnancy. These behaviors include tobacco, alcohol, and drug use as well as failure to take prenatal supplements including folic acid. According to the Centers for Disease Control and Prevention (CDC), 16% of women whose pregnancies were unplanned smoked while pregnant; in contrast, only 10% of women whose pregnancies were planned smoked during pregnancy.

Women's stress levels increase with unintended pregnancies. When faced with such a situation, a woman must make difficult decisions, including weighing her options in terms of abortion, adoption, or raising a child. Economic circumstances affect these decisions, and limited economic resources lead to more stress for women with unintended pregnancies. Recent studies have shown that the mental health of people who can become pregnant and give birth often suffers because of unintended pregnancies. Rates of postpartum depression among women with unplanned pregnancies are more than double the rates of those with planned pregnancies. Moreover, women with unintended pregnancies have elevated rates of long-term depression. At twelve months after birth, women with unwanted or mistimed pregnancies demonstrate double the rates of depression compared to women with wanted or expected pregnancies.

Some of the effects of unintended pregnancy are harder to discern and are related to larger social and educational factors. A significant effect of unintended pregnancy on American women, for example, is that they are more likely to stay with an abusive partner than those women who do not become pregnant. Unintended pregnancy, then, can contribute to the persistence of intimate partner violence. Adolescents who give birth after an unintended pregnancy are far less likely to complete high school or attend college than teens who do not give birth. Unintended pregnancy thus has a clearly negative effect on young women's educational aspirations and thus on their future employability and economic stability.

The links between maternal mortality rates and unintended pregnancy are also noteworthy. In fact, the United States has alarmingly elevated maternal mortality rates—among the highest in the developed world. These rates have been increasing in recent decades; in 1987, there were 7.2 deaths per 100,000 live births, but by 2015, that ratio had grown to 17.2 deaths per 100,000 births. Scholars are examining the relationship between these high mortality rates and the United States' elevated levels of unintended pregnancy. We know that shorter intervals between pregnancies lead to increased health risks. Mistimed or unplanned pregnancies, then, can threaten the health and well-being of people who can become pregnant.

The effects of unintended pregnancies on fetuses, infants, and children are also important to discuss. Currently, most researchers agree that there is a clear relationship between unintended pregnancies and premature birth rates. There are also links between spontaneous miscarriage and birth intention, and some evidence suggests that babies born after an unintended pregnancy have higher rates of congenital anomalies. Infants born to women with unintended pregnancies are, on average, two-thirds more likely to have low birthweights. Like maternal mortality rates, infant mortality rates in the United States are alarmingly high, particularly compared to other developed countries, and the relationship between unintended pregnancies and infant mortality rates is a current topic of research. Most studies on pregnancy intention and breastfeeding have concluded that infants born of unintended pregnancies are much less likely to be breastfed than are children whose parents intended to become pregnant. Those women who faced unintended pregnancies and did breastfeed tended to do so for shorter intervals than did those with wanted pregnancies. This reality can have negative health effects for women and infants.

Unwanted pregnancies can result in more long-term negative effects as well. Researchers have discovered higher levels of learning disabilities in children who are the result of an unintended pregnancy, and other long-term health effects are also being researched. Again, here, there are complicated factors at work. Women who carry unintended pregnancies to term and keep the child may have more difficult economic, social, and psychological circumstances that help explain the higher rates of negative childhood health outcomes in this population.

Most experts assert that preventing unintended pregnancies is essential to improving public health. How to achieve that, however, is under debate. The American College of Obstetricians and Gynecologists (2015) recommends that increased access to long-acting reversible contraceptive (LARC) methods, notably IUDs and the implant, can have a significant impact. Overall, women who plan their pregnancies are generally more able to access health care and more likely to practice healthier lifestyle choices.

What are the health effects of unintended pregnancy on families and society?

Most expert groups in the United States and internationally agree that unintended pregnancy is one of today's most significant global public health problems. In 1995, the Committee on Unintended Pregnancy, part of the U.S. Institute of Medicine, asserted that "the consequences of unintended pregnancy are serious, imposing appreciable burdens on children, women, men, and families" (Gipson, Koenig, & Hindin, 2008, p. 18).

Within individual families, unintended births can lead to stress and conflict. Researchers have reported strained and less satisfactory relationships between parents after an unintended pregnancy. Furthermore, infants or children who were unplanned or mistimed may endure greater levels of abuse or neglect. They may be treated in their families or communities as unwanted burdens. Within large families, the presence of numerous children or infants can result in stretched resources and less individual attention for each child. The realities of life in these families also sometimes cause older children, more commonly girls, to avoid or postpone education and instead help out with younger children or infants.

The wide-ranging effects of unintended pregnancy for families and society also include economic costs. Unintended pregnancies exacerbate already-existing vulnerabilities or disadvantages within families. For poorer families, an unintended pregnancy that results in the birth of an infant can add to economic stresses and precarity. Unintended pregnancy can also have a larger effect in terms of economic spending, the environment, human rights, and public health. The relationship between unintended pregnancies and public spending can be contested and controversial. In recent years, American taxpayers have paid about 12 billion dollars for medical care for women and infants as a result of unwanted or mistimed pregnancies. A greater focus on, and funding for, birth control can help reduce these costs. In 2010, for example, public resources devoted to birth control resulted in savings of over 13 billion dollars that otherwise would have been spent on costs related to unintended pregnancies (Guttmacher Institute, 2013).

Overpopulation, of course, remains a real concern in the early twenty-first century. For several decades, scholars have debated the causes of overpopulation and the role of unintended pregnancies and birth control in this discussion. Some researchers have pointed out the detrimental effects of overpopulation and have argued that the prevention of unintended pregnancies and, thus, access to birth control are essential in preventing some of the larger, harmful effects of overpopulation, including environmental harm and climate change. These views have historical origins. In the late 1700s, English economist Thomas Malthus argued that, in the modern world, the rate of population growth was greater than humanity's ability to produce and provide adequate food. When the population inevitably outstripped the food supply, Malthus argued, crisis—in the form of famine, disease, or even war—would occur to check or control the population. Malthus's views, popular for the next several hundred years, resulted in enhanced concern about the growing human population, leading to new movements to curb overpopulation. Within these movements, support for birth control became a topic of discussion.

In the twentieth century, overpopulation continued, largely unchecked. The world's population by 2000 exceeded six billion. This is an increase of over four million births in a century. At the same time, climate change became an unprecedented crisis. The links between birth control, overpopulation, and the environment are complicated, and not all experts agree on the meaning of the relationship between these phenomena. While some would advocate the promotion and use of contraception to combat overpopulation and thus global warming, others argue that some forms of birth control, made of latex or plastic, actually contribute to environmental waste and pollution. Moreover, some scholars and activists, concerned about reproductive coercion, the lasting legacy of eugenics, and the United States' horrific history of enforced sterilization, argue that discouraging unintended pregnancies through birth control use can uncomfortably perpetuate these racist and classist historical phenomena. This is because certain populations, notably women of color, incarcerated women, people with disabilities, immigrant women, and people with fewer economic resources, are often encouraged to use birth control, while others, especially well-off White women, are not. The racist and eugenic implications of this are clear.

Similar criticisms have been leveled at global attempts to curb fertility and thus population growth. In 2012, several international organizations, including the Bill and Melinda Gates Foundation and the United States Agency for International Development (USAID), created FP 2020, a global family planning initiative focused on preventing births in the developing world. Despite facing criticism that it was targeting the developing world and thus people of color, FP 2020 argues that family planning to curb population growth can occur while protecting and preserving the rights of individuals and avoiding coercion:

> Rights-based family planning is an approach to developing and implementing programs that aims to fulfill the rights of all individuals to choose whether, when, and how many children to have; to act on those choices through high-quality sexual and reproductive health services, information, and education; and to access those services free from discrimination, coercion, and violence. (FP 2020, 2019)

Reproductive justice advocates, however, have argued that

> while we agree that we must address the impact of climate change, environmental toxins, and overconsumption, we seek to pull the blame off of women of color and poor communities and target the true root causes—war, rapid urban planning, industrialization, and the lack of governmental and corporate accountability—that has contributed to the state of our bodies' and earth's lack of well-being and safety. (Jiménez et al., 2017, pp. 361–362)

How can birth control enhance the lives of women?

Access to and use of birth control can help women either not have children or plan and space their births. This ability enhances women's lives in numerous ways. Birth control can have positive health effects on women beyond fertility control. Millions of American women use forms of contraception, such as the OCP, not to prevent pregnancy but for other reasons. According to the Guttmacher Institute (2016), 14% of pill-users, or one and a half million women, take OCPs for noncontraceptive reasons. Some forms of contraception regulate irregular periods, shorten the length and lighten the flow of menstruation, alleviate cramps or pain, or allow women to not menstruate at all. One woman interviewed by the authors in 2016 about birth control responded: "I was on birth control from the time I was 24, maybe 23, 24, and I never had any issues with it. . . . It was, actually for me it was wonderful, it slowed down my periods, made them a lot lighter. [I] didn't have any issues with it. A lot of people say they gain weight; I never did. It was perfect. I was on the pill for over probably 15 years."

The pill, which helps some women regulate hormones, can also help control the symptoms of PCOS, PMS, and PMDD. It similarly can lessen the painful symptoms of endometriosis for some women. Use of the pill has been shown to decrease a woman's chances of getting certain forms of cancer, including uterine and ovarian cancer. Because other health conditions, such as acne and migraines, are often the result of hormones, the pill, by regulating hormones, also can help alleviate the symptoms of these conditions in some women.

LGBTQ+ people also use birth control for noncontraceptive reasons, including many of the previously stated reasons. As one interviewee described in 2018:

I was going just to the dermatologist, and they want to know about all your medications, and then they always want to know what method of contraception you're . . . *Are you doing this, are you doing that, are you doing this?* And then I was really frustrated because: I'm on birth control because I have PCOS, not because I'm trying to prevent pregnancy. . . . But it was like, trying to explain this to this woman was like unbelievable, 'cause you can't mix certain medications, or certain medications that they wanted to put you on, you could not get pregnant, because it was too much of a risk for the baby. It was just stupid. It's a stupid story, but I was just like, *I don't know how else. . . . Why is this always so difficult?* I'm on birth control, but it's not because I'm trying to prevent pregnancy. I don't know. I just feel like so many of the healthcare providers need more training in dealing with LGBT people.

In addition, according to recent studies, transgender or nonbinary youths who were classified as female at birth increasingly use IUDs not only for birth control but also to suppress menstruation (Akgul, Bonny, Ford, Holland-Hall, & Chelvakumar, 2019).

Birth control contributes to people's overall sexual health and well-being. As Maas and Lefkowiz (2015) summarize, "the World Health Organization defines sexual health as a state of physical, emotional, mental, and social well-being in relation to sexuality; it is not merely the absence of disease, dysfunction, or infirmity" (p. 795). It is therefore significant that recent studies demonstrate how women's sexual well-being, including sexual esteem, is enhanced by birth control. Women of all ages, but particularly adolescents or young adults, report more sexual satisfaction and pleasure when they use birth control. Contraceptive use can also alleviate the guilt, anxiety, and fear that some associate with sexual activity that may lead to unintended pregnancy.

The effects of contraception on people's lives transcend the fields of medicine or health. In fact, birth control can increase women's access to education and paid labor and thus may lead to increased earning power. Women's access to reliable, available, and effective birth control is essential to their economic stability and success. Scholars have argued that birth control can even help reduce the pay gap for women. Freed from the cycle of repeated pregnancies and births and able to plan their reproductive lives, women who use birth control have more control over their bodies and lives. They therefore may experience less stress and anxiety associated with feelings of powerlessness. Indeed, a 2012 Guttmacher study that surveyed over 2,000 American women revealed that an overwhelming majority of women believe that contraception has positively affected their lives. More than 50% of survey-takers "said that using birth control to prevent pregnancy has definitely 'allowed me to support myself financially' (56%), 'helped me to stay in school or finish my education' (51%) or 'helped me to get or keep my job or have a career' (50%)" (Frost & Lindberg, 2013, p. 467).

How does birth control enhance family, community, and societal well-being?

Controlling unintended pregnancies through birth control use and education can have transformative effects on families and societies, resulting in greater economic stability, improved health, and family stability. According to the CDC, birth control is one of the most significant public health achievements of the twentieth century. Since the early twentieth century, due in part to increased access to modern methods of birth control (see Chapter 2 of this volume), fertility rates in the United States have declined. Most people have chosen to have fewer children in the past 100 years or so. As a result, infant and child mortality rates have declined (CDC, 1999).

Birth control offers people the opportunity to plan and space births or avoid them altogether. It empowers women and increases access to educational and professional opportunities. Birth control also is foundational to the well-being of families. Indeed, the economic well-being of many families is directly related to the availability and use of contraception. Unintended pregnancies that result in the birth of children may negatively affect a family's economic stability. Already vulnerable and marginalized groups, including people of color, LGBTQ+ individuals, immigrants, and poorer women, are particularly affected by the negative financial effects of unintended pregnancy. The potential economic effects of birth control, therefore, are worth discussing. People's access to reliable, available, and effective birth control is essential to their economic stability and success.

Birth control also has the ability to enhance community well-being. Since hormonal forms of birth control became widely available in the 1970s, with women thus gaining greater control over fertility, educational opportunities and achievements for many have increased. "Between 1970 and 2012, the percent of women 25 and older with at least a high school diploma increased from 55% to 88%, and the percent with at least a bachelor's degree increased from 8% to 31%" (Kaye, Gootman, Ng, & Finley, 2014, p. 4).

There are numerous social and communal benefits of birth control. Some methods of birth control prevent the transmission of sexually transmitted infections (STIs) and thus can positively affect the health of numerous individuals and add to the well-being of families and communities. It is important to note that abstinence, condoms, and female condoms are the only methods that both provide birth control and prevent STIs; none of the other birth control methods discussed in this book prevent STIs. The United States has the highest rate of STIs among developed nations. Most of these infections occur in young people (aged 15–24). Common STIs include chlamydia, trichomoniasis, HIV, human papillomavirus (HPV), genital herpes, and hepatitis C. Since 2006, there has been a vaccine available to prevent 6 HPV-related cancers and genital warts. Chlamydia, a bacterial infection, is the most common notifiable STI in the United States today and can be easily cured. STIs are spread through all forms of sexual contact—vaginal, anal, and oral. Using a condom during these practices can help prevent the transmission of STIs as well as protect against unwanted pregnancy.

What is reproductive justice?

The 1994 International Conference on Population and Development (ICPD) in Cairo, Egypt, emerged as a turning point in women's reproductive health. For the first time, the United Nations described reproductive rights as human rights. According to the United Nations' 1948 Universal Declaration of Human Rights, all people have the right to "life, liberty and the security of person." The ICPD established that women's human rights depended on their ability to determine if, when, and how to have children. In addition, the conference recognized that women's reproductive health depended on efforts to establish gender equality and women's empowerment, as well as access to family planning services. At this transformational international moment for human rights, a group of African American women in the United States met in Chicago and established the reproductive justice movement to address the needs of women of color and other marginalized women who were largely overlooked by traditional women's rights movements, which were dominated by middle-class White women.

African American women in the United States have historically been the most effective change advocates for the health and well-being of women, children, and transgender people. In 1983, Spelman College in Atlanta hosted the first National Conference on Black Women's Health Issues. Some scholars argue that the first organization dedicated to the principles of reproductive justice, the National Black Women's Health Project, emerged from this conference. In 1997, SisterSong brought together the first national, multiethic reproductive justice collective. Today, local, regional, and national women-of-color–led organizations, including SisterSong, remain at the forefront of the movement. According to SisterSong (n.d.), reproductive justice is "the human right to maintain personal bodily autonomy, have children, not have children, and parent the children we have in safe and sustainable communities." Reproductive justice is grounded in human rights and demands bodily and reproductive autonomy for all people.

Although reproductive justice is broader than reproductive health, reproductive rights, and family planning, it provides an excellent framework to understand how systems shape women's access to and decision-making about birth control. Women's perceptions of contraception are shaped by their historical, social, and technological experiences. In interviews with women in South Carolina, one woman described family planning as a privilege, not a right. Through interviews, women described the complex ways that biological, economic, social, and political contexts influenced their ability to plan their families. Colonialism, White supremacy, and capitalism impacted their reproductive autonomy. In particular, these systems created modern, professional medicine, which pathologized women's bodies and cleaved women's ways of knowing from their families and communities. Women described barriers to family planning resulting directly from these systems, including costs (e.g., financial, emotional, time, relationship, etc.) of a yearly appointment with a health-care provider and filling a prescription at the pharmacy every month. These challenges were exacerbated for women based on factors such as race, sexual orientation, age, socioeconomic position, immigration status, ability, and geography/location.

According to Ross and Solinger (2017), reproductive justice is a framework for understanding the experience of reproduction. These scholars argue that reproductive health, including fertility management, childbirth, and parenting are fundamental human rights. As such, governments must provide access to the basic necessities required to ensure that parents can raise their children in a safe and healthy environment, which necessitates housing, fair wages and equal pay, education, high-quality health care, and freedom from violence. Without this social safety net, reproductive justice is unattainable. This approach highlights the needs of marginalized communities and communities of color facing individual, societal, and systemic challenges to health and well-being. To protect women from forced reproduction, as well as coerced suppression of fertility and sterilization, reproductive justice advocates for improvements to systems of health care, immigration, and incarceration (Ross & Solinger, 2017).

A reproductive justice approach ensures that women maintain the right to decide if, when, and how to become a parent. This includes access to comprehensive sex education, fertility management, STI prevention and treatment, prenatal and pregnancy care, and choices in childbirth. The Center for Reproductive Rights stresses that all women have the right to benefit from scientific progress. Women and couples deserve knowledge of and access to reproductive technologies, ranging from contraception, egg freezing, in vitro fertilization, and surrogacy (Sundstrom, 2015). Benefiting from scientific progress also means understanding the risks of medicalized reproduction, including prenatal testing and cesarean section, for example. As a result, knowledge of and equal access to contraception is one of the fundamental elements of reproductive justice.

How do factors such as race/ethnicity, class/socioeconomic position, ability, age, gender/sexuality, and immigration status influence reproductive oppression and social inequality?

Grounding reproductive justice in women's fundamental human rights moves reproductive freedom beyond individualist notions of choice to a collective understanding of the intersectionality of access to reproductive health. In other words, without access to reproductive health, there can be no choice. According to Kimala Price, this framework connects reproductive health and rights with other social justice issues, such as education, poverty, housing, economic justice, environmental justice, immigration policy, prisoners' rights, drug policies, and violence. Violence includes individual forms of violence, such as intimate partner violence, as well as institutional and state-sponsored violence. Institutional violence that impacts women's reproductive health may include policies that reflect colonialism, White supremacy, neoliberalism, criminalization, and capitalism. Reproductive justice seeks to dismantle the systems, policies, and dimensions of social inequality that oppress and restrict reproductive rights.

Reproductive justice centers on the lived experiences of marginalized women, especially women of color. In the United States, the history of slavery, forced reproduction, and coercive government policies (discussed in Chapter 2 of this volume), continues to impact African American women's reproductive decision-making. Government and institutional policies have targeted women of color to control their fertility, either to force or prevent women from having children. Population control initiatives grounded in racist ideologies have promoted immigration restrictions, welfare reform, sterilization, and targeted family planning. These policies are disproportionately aimed at women of color to control their reproductive health and rights; in this context, women of color have been prescient in linking civil rights with reproductive rights. Even when African American nationalist leaders promoted pronatalism, African American women supported reproductive freedom and access to family planning services. Today, decision-making about birth control continues to be impacted by a legacy of coercion.

How does birth control fit within reproductive justice?

Equal access to contraception is necessary to achieve reproductive justice. The reproductive justice framework illustrates how systems shape women's access to and decision-making about birth control. Policies that provide incentives for the use of certain contraceptive methods have been overturned due to concerns about coercive and unethical influence on women's contraceptive decision-making. However, research shows that health-care providers continue to display individual bias based on patients' markers of difference (e.g., race/ethnicity, socioeconomic position) that impact their contraceptive recommendations. Health-care providers may be more likely to recommend a LARC method to a woman of color and may be more likely to resist removing such methods when patients are dissatisfied. Studies show that women who are publicly insured through programs such as Medicaid are more likely to use LARC methods or female sterilization compared to women with private health insurance. This suggests that low-income women and women of color are perceived differently by health-care providers and that they may receive contraceptive recommendations based on providers' stereotypes rather than their own needs, preferences, and values. Indeed, women themselves report perceived discrimination based on race/ethnicity, socioeconomic position, and gender that impacts their contraceptive method decision-making and use.

Women in the United States must interact with the health-care system and individual health-care providers to access the most effective methods of birth control. These same systems and individuals may limit some women's autonomy in contraceptive decision-making. Health-care providers may fail to provide a range of contraceptive options or persuade certain women to use particular methods of contraception without considering their individual needs. Coercion occurs when health-care providers offer different recommendations or resist patient preferences because of assumptions based on patient characteristics, including gender, race/ethnicity, socioeconomic position, immigration status, ability, sexual orientation, and age. Overemphasizing certain methods of contraception without considering underlying biological, economic, social, and political contexts limits women's bodily and reproductive autonomy.

What are the popular perceptions of contraception?

Birth control is a fact of life, integral to most people's lives and daily experiences. The vast majority of Americans support birth control and contraception. In a 2018 survey conducted by Power to Decide, "nearly 8 in 10 (78%) adults in the United States—including 66% of Republicans and 93% of Democrats—consider[ed] birth control to be a basic part of women's health care" (Power to Decide, 2018). The same survey demonstrated that over 80% of people favored increased access to birth control for all women, including adolescents, and about 75% supported the idea that local and state governments, as well as the federal government, should fund birth control for adult women (Power to Decide, 2018). Even those who consider themselves to be religious are overwhelmingly in favor of birth control. Of sexually active women who define themselves as Christian (Catholic or Protestant), 99% have used a form of contraception. One woman we interviewed in 2016, who was in her 60s at the time, responded to the question: What comes to mind when you hear the words "contraception" or "birth control"? with one word: "Necessary." Another interviewee, a 67-year old woman, responded to the same question with another equally meaningful word: "Amen."

How does media portrayal of birth control impact how it is used?

American women have learned about family planning through community education programs, health-care providers, friends and family, and local and mass media. In our interviews, women reported that they received information about birth control from all of these sources. Some women told us that they were cautious about believing information that came from the media; others affirmed that the most important opinions that influenced their understandings of birth control were those of doctors, friends, and family. In our interviews, a woman's age sometimes determined her perceptions about contraception. Some women over age 50, for example, perhaps because of their memories of the Dalkon Shield controversy, believed that the IUD was not only dangerous but may not even be available today. According to one woman, ". . . the IUD, I heard it can mess up or something, I don't want that to happen so I'd like to know how others [reacted to the IUD], not to compare myself, but just to make sure I'm safe."

The news media, locally and nationally, influences which issues are covered and how the issues are presented. Through the powerful role of agenda-setting, mass media chooses which issues receive coverage and attention. Through framing, the media influences how individuals think about certain issues. Research shows that health information in the mass media may be misleading based on how the issue is framed. Reporters might fail to cover a topic sufficiently or at all, provide too much or too little information, or include misinformation or false equivalency. The news media continues to play a critical role in how women understand and think about birth control.

In the early nineteenth century, women and midwives knew how to prevent pregnancy and shared this information openly. According to Parry (2013), in the mid-1800s, newspapers and magazines included advertisements for drugs and home remedies to prevent pregnancy. In an effort to discredit midwives and solidify the newly established obstetrician–gynecologist profession, however, medical professionals joined moral purity campaigners to outlaw advertising of contraception and abortion. The Comstock Act of 1873 prohibited the distribution of materials about contraception. Margaret Sanger and birth control advocates resisted the Comstock law's intent to silence women by developing strategies to attract mass media coverage. Through the strategic use of mass media, birth control received support and acceptance, transitioning from a private issue to a public topic that could be discussed openly. In 1914, Sanger published the *Family Limitation* pamphlet to openly defy and challenge the Comstock law. This dissent received widespread mass media coverage, and many women learned about birth control through the news.

The Comstock law remained in place until 1965 when *Griswold vs. Connecticut* ruled in favor of a person's right to privacy, finding it was unconstitutional to restrict access to birth control. However, contraceptive advertising was banned by the National Association of Broadcasters until 1982. After the ban's repeal, broadcasters avoided advertising contraception, fearing backlash from vocal conservative special interest groups. The American Academy of Pediatrics released a policy statement in 1995 arguing that media leaders have a responsibility to provide information about contraception. Today, numerous public health campaigns provide information about birth control, including Power to Decide's #ThxBirth Control and Bedsider.org campaigns and MTV's It's Your (Sex) Life campaign. There is a growing need for health communicators to present the harms and benefits of contraception in the context of women's lived experiences.

What is "contraceptive scare"?

While some popular perceptions of contraception are accurate, others are not— and may even be harmful. In the United States, some media outlets perpetuate misinformation or encourage fear-mongering in matters related to reproductive health. One way that media outlets skew women's understanding of risk is by reporting relative measures of risk and seldomly presenting comprehensive information about absolute risk (Jensen & Trussell, 2012). Relative measures of risk are often expressed as percentages and fail to convey the chance of something happening. Absolute risk presents whole numbers that help accurately communicate the true impact or size of the risk. Scholars argue that presenting baseline risks and reporting absolute risk is more accurate than relative risk and helps to support patient-centered medical decision-making. Experts suggest that relative risks are more likely to be misunderstood and to be misleading.

"Contraceptive scare" is a term used to describe the reality that some people perceive a link between contraception and adverse health effects (even while pregnancy and childbirth are in fact far more risky to women's health than birth control). For healthy nonsmoking women, the pill offers a 240 times lower risk of death than do pregnancy complications (Becker & Betstadt, 2013). Still, many people continue to believe that birth control is dangerous and linked to health problems such as cancer, infertility, and blood clots. Historical examples also affect women's views of contraception today. In the 1970s, for example, problems with the Dalkon Shield, a kind of IUD, resulted in lasting suspicion of this particular birth control method. The Dalkon Shield came on the market in the early 1970s as one of dozens of IUD devices. Because it was not a drug or medication, it did not undergo serious testing by the U.S. Food and Drug Administration (FDA). By 1974, over 2.5 million American women were using the Dalkon Shield. It was removed from the market that same year, however, when it was discovered that it had caused thousands of women to contract pelvic inflammatory disease. Ultimately, the Dalkon Shield led to 17 deaths and over 200,000 infections and miscarriages (Bahr, 2012).

Boonstra and colleagues (2000) described the "boom and bust" phenomenon of contraceptive technology. When new contraceptive methods are introduced, media tend to focus on the benefits and potential of the new contraception, often downplaying limitations or side effects. This leads to a boom or increase in uptake. When media highlight sensational stories of side effects and complications, often omitting or burying substantive context, this leads to a bust or dramatic decline in use. In *New York Magazine*, Eric Pooley described the media's approach as, "if it bleeds, it leads." For example, a 2014 *Vanity Fair* article by Marie Brenner, "Danger in the Ring" posed a deceptive question, "Is the contraceptive NuvaRing killing thousands?" Although the publication advertised a "full investigation," the article offered fear-mongering anecdotes with questionable sources and no scientific evidence. Media attention spotlighting the limitations of contraceptive methods often results in a bust or contraceptive scare, prompting women to discontinue use and leading to more unintended pregnancies. The boom-and-bust cycle juxtaposes a "perfect method" of contraception with sensationalized side effects and limitations. Without substantive analysis, news coverage of contraception undermines an accurate understanding of the pros and cons of contraceptive methods.

Media stories about the risk of contraception also tend to omit the risks of pregnancy and childbirth. The popular press downplays the risks of pregnancy and childbirth, favoring a narrative that modern medicine can protect women and infants. In fact, studies show that the use of any contraceptive method prevents deaths related to pregnancy and childbirth. A recent study found that approximately half of women incorrectly thought that hormonal contraception is more dangerous than pregnancy based on misunderstandings of the risk of pulmonary embolism, cancer, and infertility (Becker & Betstadt, 2013). These results may be attributed to the impact of contraceptive scare on women's understanding of contraception.

The boom-and-bust phenomenon may also help explain women's unmet need for contraception related to a lack of innovation. First in 1970 and again in 1989, chemist Carl Djerassi, who has been called the father of the pill, described the stagnation of contraceptive research and development. He correctly predicted that only minor modifications would be made to nineteenth and twentieth century methods of birth control. Djerassi (1989) identified the increase of medical litigation in the United States, the impact of Senator Nelson's 1970 congressional hearing about the safety of the pill, the Dalkon Shield IUD, and the FDA's testing requirements as the main reasons limiting development of new and innovative methods of contraception. In 1969, journalist Barbara Seaman released *The Doctor's Case Against the Pill*, which included anecdotes from women and health-care providers. This book served as a catalyst for the Nelson congressional hearings on the safety of the pill. The media coverage of these events led women to discontinue the pill in the short term and strongly impacted women's perspectives of contraceptive safety (Boonstra et al., 2000).

As we described earlier in this chapter, the Dalkon Shield was a malfunctioning IUD that increased the risk of pelvic inflammatory disease and infertility. The manufacturer voluntarily discontinued sale of the IUD in 1974 because of problems with the design and manufacture of the product. Although the risk was limited to the Dalkon Shield, media coverage failed to distinguish between different IUDs. This led to an immediate and long-term discontinuation of the IUD among women in the United States (Boonstra et al., 2000). Although rates of IUD use have increased modestly in recent years, American women choose the IUD less frequently than women in other countries, which may be attributed to sensational and incomplete media coverage of the Dalkon Shield.

Women also receive one-sided and incomplete information from pharmaceutical advertisements and commercials paid for by personal injury lawyers. Women we have talked with suggested that the complications listed in lawsuit commercials were a source of concern. These women summarized the takeaway message from these ads, "Mirena® could have done this to you" and "If you or a loved one has even died . . ." Bayer's "beyond birth control" campaign for the oral contraceptive Yaz® was cited by the FDA for false advertising because it failed to clearly distinguish an indication to treat PMDD, which did not cover PMS. Personal injury lawyers pay for commercials to recruit women who believe they have experienced negative health effects because of hormonal contraception. Thousands of lawsuits have been filed to seek monetary compensation based on perceived injuries related to the use of IUDs, OCPs, implants, patches, and rings. Increasingly, lawyers and health activists are connecting with patient advocacy groups online. Lindheim and colleagues (2019) described how Essure®, a permanent hysteroscopic sterilization device that offered many benefits compared to traditional tubal ligation surgery, was pulled from the market in 2018 based largely on the advocacy of a Facebook group that became Advocating Safety in Healthcare E-Sisters (ASHES) and the Netflix documentary, "The Bleeding Edge." Although social media offers the potential to raise the voices of vulnerable women who may not otherwise be heard, it also poses a risk to those same women who may be targeted by organized movements and individuals who seek to profit from their health outcomes.

Coverage of contraceptive methods in the popular press and scientific literature leads to contraceptive scare and the boom and bust phenomenon. Contraceptive scare impacts women's perceptions of hormonal contraception and the risk of negative health effects. This cycle limits women's choices of contraception. Women in the United States have fewer contraceptive options and are less likely to choose LARC options than women in other countries. Sensationalized media coverage of contraception has led women to discontinue some methods of contraception, resulting in increased unintended pregnancies. Women and couples have demonstrated unmet contraception need. This may be attributed in part to sensationalized media coverage of contraception risks.

2

WHAT IS BIRTH CONTROL?

How does birth control work?

Most people who can become pregnant and give birth menstruate and ovulate. Menstruation is more commonly known as a "period" and refers to monthly vaginal bleeding that is a normal part of the menstrual cycle for most women. In the United States today, most girls or adolescents start menstruating ("menarche") between the ages of 11 and 15. For girls and women who have passed menarche, every month the body prepares itself for pregnancy. The hormones estrogen and progesterone, which are located in the ovaries, get ready for a potential pregnancy each month by causing build-up on the lining of the uterus. This occurs in case a fertilized egg attaches to the lining of the uterus, resulting in a pregnancy. If no fertilized egg attaches to the uterine lining, however, then the build-up on the lining is expelled. This usually occurs each month, resulting in menstruation. An image of the female reproductive system is pictured in Figure 2.1.

Ovulation is when an egg, located in a person's ovary, exits the ovary and travels through the fallopian tubes. This usually happens approximately once a month. An unfertilized egg is usually viable for up to 24 hours. Pregnancy happens if sperm, usually ejaculated from a man's penis, encounters an egg during this time and fertilizes the egg. Inside a woman's body,

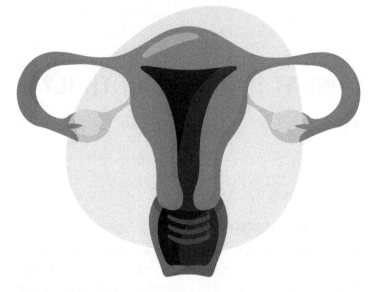

Figure 2.1. The Female Reproductive System.

sperm can live for up to five days. If a fertilized egg implants in the lining of the uterus (a process that can take several days), that person becomes pregnant.

Birth control attempts to prevent pregnancy. It works differently depending on the chosen method. The specific methods available are discussed in more detail later in this chapter. When using behavioral methods, such as abstinence, coitus interruptus (withdrawal before ejaculation), and fertility awareness methods including natural family planning, people seek to adjust, control, or alter their behavior to prevent pregnancy. Barrier methods, which include condoms and diaphragms, are physical barriers placed either on the man's penis or in the woman's vagina, sometimes covering her cervix. These barriers block the sperm from getting to the egg and thus prevent fertilization. Substances such as spermicides work by damaging sperm, which then cannot travel as well to fertilize an egg. Permanent methods of birth control, including both male and female sterilization, involve an operation that alters a person's anatomy and makes it impossible for sperm and/or an egg to travel and meet each other.

Hormonal methods of birth control are usually categorized into two groups: short-acting methods (such as the birth control pill, patch, and shot) and long-acting reversible contraception or LARC (such as the intrauterine device [IUD] or implant). These methods produce hormones such as estrogen and/or progestin. Estrogen is a hormone produced in the ovaries. Progestin is a synthetic form of the natural hormone progesterone. Estrogen and progesterone/progestin affect menstruation and fertility. When used in hormonal forms of birth control, they prevent a woman's ovaries from releasing eggs (ovulation). Some hormonal methods of birth control also make it difficult for sperm to reach an egg by thickening a woman's cervical mucus. In addition, hormonal methods may prevent the potential implantation of a fertilized egg in the uterus by thinning the lining of the uterus.

What are the different methods of birth control available today?

When asked about the methods of birth control available, women we interviewed in 2016 had a variety of responses. As one stated, "I know the patch, um, condoms, of course, and, um, the pills, the shots, the IUD, and, um, there's some more I can't remember but I know there's a lot. Diaphragm, I don't know if they still use that or not." Another woman, who was in her 60s, responded:

Some of them probably are outdated just because of my age. But I know about the pill, I know about the shot, there's some ring, I know about the IUD, I don't know if people use that anymore, there was a sponge when I was coming around. Then condoms, and then the old pull-out method. So those are pretty much my. . . . There was

film. A VC something film that came around when I was
in my 20s. I remember trying that.

As these narratives suggest, there are a variety of birth control methods available in the United States, and some of these
have been around for decades. Behavioral methods, fertility
awareness methods, barrier methods, hormonal methods, and
permanent methods are all readily accessible today.

Abstinence means avoiding heterosexual vaginal sexual intercourse (penile–vaginal penetration). Without this kind of
sexual activity, there is little chance for a sperm and an egg to
meet. Abstinence must be practiced consistently to be effective. Coitus interruptus, another behavioral method, is withdrawal of the penis from the vagina before ejaculation. Coitus
interruptus may work in some cases by preventing contact between a sperm and an egg; however, this method is far from
foolproof because some semen usually comes out of the penis
before ejaculation. This pre-ejaculate can cause pregnancy.

Fertility awareness methods also require regulating behavior. Women who follow this path attempt to understand their
monthly fertility patterns to discern when they are ovulating
and thus to determine the days when they are likely fertile
(usually around six days per month). They practice periodic
abstinence, avoiding intercourse on days when they are potentially fertile and restricting penile–vaginal penetrative sex to
days of the month when conception is unlikely. What is usually
called the "rhythm method" involves monitoring a woman's
monthly cycle and attempting to determine her number of
fertile days based on that cycle. Most women ovulate around
day 14 of their monthly cycle. Once a woman determines her
average monthly cycle, she can then avoid intercourse for several days before and after day 14. Another family planning
method is the basil body temperature method. Most women's
temperatures rise upon ovulation, so taking a woman's temperature every day can help discern when ovulation occurs.

Avoiding sexual intercourse on days when a woman has an elevated temperature may help prevent pregnancy. Lastly, the cervical mucus method can be used. Here, a woman monitors her vaginal discharge and mucus. This mucus becomes slippery and stretchy (like the texture of an egg white) during ovulation; therefore, avoiding sexual intercourse when the cervical mucus assumes this texture may help prevent pregnancy as well.

The lactational amenorrhea method is one that some breastfeeding women use. It can be effective under the following conditions: when a woman has given birth less than six months previously, she is breastfeeding exclusively and frequently, and she is not menstruating (a condition called "amenorrhea"). Under these circumstances, breastfeeding causes an excess of a hormone called prolactin. The prolactin, in turn, lessens the production of estrogen and prevents ovulation. Without ovulation, no egg leaves the ovary to travel through the fallopian tubes. Intercourse during this time, therefore, may not result in conception.

Barrier methods, which block the sperm from getting to the egg and thus prevent fertilization and the creation of an embryo, are accessible and popular in the United States. Most commonly known and used is the male condom. Worn on a man's penis during intercourse, a condom prevents sperm from entering a woman's body and fertilizing an egg. Most male condoms today are made of latex or polyisoprene, and in addition to being effective forms of birth control, they also protect against most sexually transmitted infections (STIs), including human immunodeficiency virus (HIV). Condoms are available over the counter at most drug stores or pharmacies. They are not covered by health insurance plans. They are disposable and only can be used once. Condoms come in different shapes, sizes, and textures; some are flavored. There are dozens of brands of male condoms available, including Trojan® and Durex®.

A female condom, sometimes also known as an "internal" condom, is worn by a woman. Made of plastic, it is inserted into the vagina and, like the male condom, provides a physical barrier that prevents sperm from reaching an egg. Like the male condom, the female condom is not covered by health insurance plans and protects against most forms of STIs. In the United States, the brand of female condom sold is the FC2 Female Condom®.

Usually made of silicone, a diaphragm is a cup-shaped or bowl-shaped barrier that is placed deep inside the vagina before sexual intercourse to cover the cervix. With the cervix covered, sperm are not able to travel to an egg. Diaphragms, marketed in the United States under the name Caya®, frequently are used with spermicide, a chemical that makes it difficult for sperm to move. A cervical cap, sold as FemCap® in the United States, is a small cup that covers the cervix and prevents fertilization. It is similar to a diaphragm but is generally smaller and may be left in for a longer period of time after intercourse. Diaphragms and cervical caps must be fitted to your body by a physician and thus are only available in the United States via prescription. Like diaphragms and cervical caps, contraceptive sponges are placed in the vagina, covering the cervix, before sexual intercourse. To be effective, the sponge must remain in the vagina for approximately six hours after intercourse. Then it can be removed and disposed of. The only brand of contraceptive sponge available in the United States is the Today® sponge.

Spermicides, which can be gels, foams, or film, are available over the counter in most drug stores in the United States. Brand names include Contceptrol®, Emko®, Delfen Foam®, Prochive®, and Advantage-S®. Spermicides are chemical substances that take the form of a gel, cream, lotion, suppository, foam, or film (vaginal contraceptive film). Placed deep in the vagina before sex (ideally at least 15 to 20 minutes before intercourse), the chemicals in these substances help impede the movement of sperm and thus may prevent the sperm from fertilizing an egg.

Most spermicides don't actually kill sperm; rather, they prevent sperm from moving effectively. Some spermicides also help create a barrier to block the cervix so that sperm cannot enter and fertilize an egg. Spermicides are used on their own as well as in conjunction with diaphragms, cervical caps, and sponges.

Short-acting hormonal methods include the oral contraceptive pill (OCP) or birth control pill, the mini-pill, the patch, the shot, and the vaginal ring. LARC methods provide lasting contraception without the need for significant user initiative. They include hormonal and nonhormonal IUDs, which are small plastic T-shaped devices that are inserted into the uterus, and the contraceptive implant, which is a small rod inserted into a woman's arm.

OCPs, usually taken orally one a day, work by releasing hormones into the body. Most OCPs contain two hormones: progestin and estrogen. The "mini-pill," however, only contains the hormone progestin. The injection Depo-Provera®, which contains progestin, is given to a woman by a doctor every three months or so. The transdermal contraceptive patch, sold under the name Xulane®, is a skin patch that a woman wears on her body (usually the abdomen or buttocks), replacing it every three weeks or so. It releases the hormones progestin and estrogen into the bloodstream. The hormonal vaginal contraceptive ring, called NuvaRing®, similarly releases progestin and estrogen into the body; however, the ring uses a lower dose of hormones than other methods, which may result in fewer side effects. The ring is placed inside the vagina for approximately three weeks and then must be replaced. This is a self-controlled method of birth control and does not require a health-care provider to insert or demonstrate how to put it in. There is no exact position it needs to be in—as long as it is in comfortably, it is working.

LARC methods work more effectively and for longer periods of time. The contraceptive implant, Nexplanon®, is a small rod-like flexible device that is inserted under the skin of a woman's upper arm. It can remain there and work effectively for up to three years. The implant works by releasing the hormone progestin into a woman's body. Today, there are a plethora of IUDs on the American market. IUDs are small, T-shaped devices made out of plastic or copper. Most IUDs, except for the ParaGard® copper IUD, release hormones. IUDs are inserted by a physician, who places the IUD inside a woman's uterus. The Mirena® IUD, which is approved by the U.S. Food and Drug Administration (FDA) not only for pregnancy prevention but also to treat heavy menstrual bleeding, is made of flexible plastic. It can be left in the body and remain effective for five to seven years. The Liletta® IUD is a less expensive option that is FDA approved for use up to three years. Skyla® is known as a "mini-IUD," and it is approved for use up to three years with marketing aimed at women who have not yet had children. Like Mirena®, it contains hormones, but Skyla® has less progestin than Mirena®, and it is smaller. Another hormonal IUD, Kyleena®, also is available for women and lasts up to five years. These IUDs may not be effective until approximately one week after insertion, so a back-up method of contraception should be used during that time. The ParaGard® IUD is an IUD that contains no hormones. Instead, it is wrapped in copper; the copper is toxic to sperm. The ParaGard® IUD is effective in preventing pregnancy immediately after insertion and can also be used as emergency contraception (see the following discussion). It can be left in place for up to 10 years. LARC methods must be prescribed by a physician. New studies show that many of these methods may be effective for longer periods of time.

Sterilization consists of a medical procedure to permanently prevent conception from taking place, although some forms of sterilization may be surgically reversible. Male sterilization or vasectomy involves cutting the vas deferens. This prevents sperm from getting into semen. In the female sterilization procedure known as tubal ligation, physicians usually cut and tie the fallopian tubes so that the egg is not able to leave the ovary and travel to meet a sperm and therefore fertilization will not be possible. It also prevents the sperm from traveling and meeting an egg. Both vasectomies and tubal ligations must be performed by a physician in a hospital or clinic, although both are usually outpatient surgeries. Hysterectomies and oophorectomies, in which the uterus or ovaries are surgically removed, also are permanent methods of birth control performed by a physician in a hospital.

What are hormonal methods of birth control?

Hormonal birth control methods release either progestin or both estrogen and progestin into a woman's body. Most hormonal birth control methods require a physician's prescription.

What are nonhormonal methods of birth control?

Nonhormonal methods of birth control include behavioral modification methods, barrier methods, and permanent sterilization.

What are the most commonly used methods of birth control?

Figure 2.2 lists, in order, the most popular forms of birth control in the United States as of 2019. It includes usage rates, failure rates, and images of the methods.

The method of birth control that individuals use depends on a variety of factors. In our research, women who were asked about their preferred methods of birth control cited several important factors in their contraceptive decision-making (Gazit, 2003). The following were the most common: (a) effectiveness, (b) ease or convenience, (c), comfort, (d) low risk of side effects, and (e) cost. As one woman explained, "the outcome, the effectiveness, that's the most important thing. And how convenient is it? How comfortable is it?" When an interviewer asked another woman, "What do you think women want when they are choosing a type of birth control?" the woman responded, "I guess they just want easy . . . mostly and something that wouldn't, like, have a side effect." Additional factors, including religious beliefs or values and political views, availability of the method, and popular perceptions of the particular method may impact contraceptive choice.

Usage Rate %	Failure Rate %	Method	Image
23.5	9	Pill	
19.5	0.5	Female Sterilization	
14.6	18	Male Condom	
11.8	0.2-0.8	IUD	
8.1	22	Coitus Interruptus	
3.9	6	Injection	
2.6	0.05	Implant	
2.4	9	Vaginal Ring	
2.2	24	Fertility awareness -based methods	
>0.6	28	Spermicides	
>0.6	21	Female condom	
>0.6	12-24	Sponge	
>0.6	12	Diaphragm	
0.2	9	Patch	

Data compiled from the CDC (https://www.cdc.gov/reproductivehealth/contraception/ unintendedpregnancy/pdf/Contraceptive_methods_508.pdf)

Figure 2.2. Most Popular Forms of Birth Control in the United States.

Even though it is only about 91% effective at pregnancy prevention with typical use, the OCP or birth control pill is the most widely used form of contraception today in the United States, and it has been for decades. In fact, four out of five American women who have ever had penile–vaginal sexual intercourse have taken "the pill" at some point in their lives. In some ways, then, being "on the pill" has become synonymous with "taking birth control." In our research, when we ask women "so what comes to mind when you hear the words birth control or contraception?" many respond immediately, "The pill."

The reasons for the pill's popularity are complex. The invention of the pill in the mid-twentieth century was revolutionary for women, who now had an effective method of birth control that did not require male cooperation or even knowledge but also, unlike the diaphragm, did not require insertion before intercourse. The resulting feelings of independence, control, and confidence that women experienced should not be underestimated. According to journalist Loretta McLoughlin,

> for the very, very, very first time, women would be set free to enjoy sex, without the fear of pregnancy hanging over their head. They did not have to get up in the dark of night as one woman said and walk across the ice cold linoleum in her bare foot to go into the bathroom and get the diaphragm. Women for the very, very first time were going to be sexually as free as men. (Gatiz, 2003)

One of our research participants said of the pill in 2016, "I like knowing that it is under my control, because I'm pretty good about taking it at the same time every day and that makes me feel good about the birth control working effectively."

The support of the medical profession also bolsters the pill's popularity. Most health-care providers, when discussing contraception with their patients, particularly younger women or adolescents, emphasize the pill as the most common and perhaps best option. Moreover, some women, and particularly adolescent women, believe incorrectly that because the pill is the most commonly known, discussed, publicized, and used method of contraception, it must be the most effective method. According to one interviewee, "most people take the pill. I would think it's the most effective." Another agreed, "[LARC methods] must be less effective because they are not as popular [as the pill]."

The pill's popularity has been helped by effective and widespread marketing campaigns. Elizabeth Siegel Watkins argues that marketing plans and money-making strategies, more so than efficacy, have contributed to the pill's ubiquity. Since the 1990s especially, marketing campaigns have highlighted not only the pill's contraceptive effects but also its utility as a "lifestyle drug," which certainly has contributed to its popularity. As Watkins (2012) explains, *"lifestyle drugs* . . . generally describe medications that are designed to improve a person's quality of life by treating less serious conditions; they also have been called cosmetic, life-enhancing, recreational, or discretionary."* (p. 1464; emphasis in original) In the case of the pill, manufacturers have touted its abilities to curb acne, alleviate period pain and cramps, and regulate or stop menstruation. These marketing campaigns have been overwhelmingly successful since the late twentieth century.

In the United States, female sterilization is the second-most popular form of birth control. Chosen by 21.8% of all contraceptive users, its popularity is tied to the fact that it offers a permanent method of pregnancy prevention. It can be controversial because studies show that certain groups of women are encouraged to adopt it. As the Guttmacher Institute (2018) explains,

reliance on female sterilization varies among subgroups of women. It is most common among blacks and Hispanics, women aged 35 or older, ever-married women, women with two or more children, women living below 150% of the federal poverty level, women with less than a college education, women living outside of a metropolitan area, and those with public or no health insurance.

Thus, it is important to remember that a variety of factors contribute to the popularity of particular methods of contraception.

After the OCP and female sterilization, male condoms are the most common form of birth control. Condoms may be preferred because they are relatively inexpensive, are available without a prescription at almost all drug stores, can be used by men, and are able to be used once and then thrown away. Some birth control users think of the condom as having fewer potential side effects than other contraceptive methods. As one interviewee described,

anything that's long term, I don't want to do that. Not when it comes to a drug. Condoms for sure but not when it comes to birth control that I have to take orally or something like that that could have an adverse effect. Side effects I don't want any part of that. But a condom yeah of course, I'm all for that.

Furthermore, male condoms' popularity may be related to their multi-purpose use: they not only prevent pregnancy but also prevent the transmission of STIs.

Although experts recommend LARC methods such as the IUD and implant for their ease and effectiveness, American women are less likely to use them than are women in other parts of the developed world. In the 2000s, on average only about six to nine percent of American women had used the IUD or the implant. Some women interviewed about their birth control preferences revealed that while they were comfortable consuming a pill, they were somewhat uneasy about LARC methods. As one woman said, "I think you know, definitely something that's, um, not so invasive. You know, I think that that does make a big difference. . . . And so I think birth control pills are, you know, I think they prefer that. I think most women do, compared to something that you have inside of you." A lack of knowledge about and understanding of LARC methods contributes to its relatively low usage. Older women (women aged 60 and over) interviewed by the authors often expressed surprise at how long LARC contraceptive protections lasted. One 62-year-old woman, for example, had the following exchange with her interviewer:

INTERVIEWEE: "I wish they had all of this stuff when I was young. Back in my day people didn't really talk about it much. You know my mom never explained that to me. So you can get a shot that works for three years now?"

INTERVIEWER: "The shot works for three months but the implant works for three years."

INTERVIEWEE: "Wow. Well that's amazing."

Myths that LARC methods cause infertility or other health problems also persist. Despite the fact that IUDs in the United States today are regulated and proven to be safe and highly effective, some women still fear that they will cause negative side effects or health effects. The history of the Dalkon Shield, discussed in Chapter 1 of this volume, has tainted all IUDs in the minds of some, older women in particular. Because these women often council their daughters about contraception, they may pass on negative impressions of IUDs. Younger women often rely on the advice and opinion of their mothers when deciding on a method of birth control, so the opinions of mothers matter (Payne, Sundstrom, & DeMaria, 2016).

Nonetheless, in recent years, the use of LARC methods has been steadily increasing. Only 2.4% of contraceptive users utilized LARC methods in 2002; by 2013, that figure had increased to 11.6%.

What is perfect use?

Perfect use is when a method of birth control is used correctly and consistently, such as in a laboratory or clinical trial setting. The result is a higher level of contraceptive protection and success. It is easier to achieve perfect use with methods of birth control that do not require active human intervention. LARC methods, for example, such as the Mirena® IUD and the implant, which are inserted once by a physician and last for several years, have almost identical perfect use and typical use rates.

What is typical use?

Typical use is a phrase used to describe how women use a contraceptive method in their everyday lives, which may not be perfectly consistent or correct. Typical use, which accounts for human error, has higher failure rates than perfect use. Methods that require human behavior modification or consistent effort, such as the OCP and the male condom, demonstrate typical use. Today, 50% of all unintended pregnancies result from inconsistent or incorrect use of contraception.

How effective are today's methods of birth control in preventing pregnancy?

The effectiveness of birth control methods varies widely. Today, the birth control methods that are most effective are sterilization and LARC methods—IUDs or the implant. Permanent methods of birth control (sterilization) have very low failure rates. The failure rates for both tubal ligation and vasectomy are less than 1%. With typical use, LARC methods also have a less than 1% failure rate. LARC methods are so effective at preventing pregnancy because (a) after insertion they do not require action on the part of a user for years at a time and (b) they can be easily and correctly inserted by a physician; user error, therefore, rarely plays a part in LARC methods.

Other methods, including short-term hormonal contraceptive methods and barrier methods, have higher typical-use failure rate than do LARC methods because they are susceptible to inconsistent use or user error. Approximately 43% of unintended pregnancies are a result of user error or inconsistent contraceptive use. The injection has a 4% failure rate, for example, while the patch and the ring both have approximately a 7% failure rate. Because it is so susceptible to human error, the OCP has a typical-use failure rate of approximately 8% to 9%. This failure rate is usually attributed to a user's forgetting to take the pill or taking it inconsistently or at different times of day.

Barrier methods have comparatively high failure rates. With typical use, the male condom has, on average, a 13% failure rate, and the female condom has a rate of approximately 21%. The typical use failure rate for the diaphragm is 17%. The sponge's failure rate is 14%, and that of the vaginal contraceptive film, 21%.

Coitus interruptus has a failure rate of approximately 20%. Fertility awareness methods, such as natural family planning or the rhythm method require people to regulate their sexual actions consistently and therefore have comparatively high failure rates—currently 24%.

What is emergency contraception or the morning-after pill?

Pregnancy does not occur immediately after sex; in fact, conception can take up to several days after penile–vaginal penetrative sexual intercourse. Unlike most of the methods of birth control discussed so far, emergency contraception (EC) can be used *after* intercourse to prevent unintended pregnancy. If a person has sex without using contraception, if their birth control method fails, or if they are raped, they may use EC in the hours and days after sex. The different forms of EC contain hormones that can prevent fertilization of an egg and can impede a fertilized egg's implantation in the lining of a woman's uterus. EC, however, will not work after implantation has occurred. EC comes in different forms. The most effective method is a ParaGard® copper IUD, which can be inserted up to 5 days after unprotected sex. The copper in the IUD harms sperm, making them less able to fertilize an egg. After being used as EC, the copper IUD may be left in for as many as 10 years and thus can double as effective long-term birth control.

EC also comes in pill form. Pills may be taken after sexual intercourse (thus the common label "morning-after pill"). There are different types of EC pills: (a) pills containing ulipristal acetate (brand name Ella®) and (b) pills containing progestin (brand names Plan B®, After Pill®, One Step®). Ulipristal pills, which release hormones that delay ovulation, are more effective, although they are only available by prescription. They can be taken effectively up to 5 days after unprotected sex. Progestin pills are less effective but are available over the counter in the United States. Most experts recommend that progestin pills be taken within 72 hours of sexual intercourse, although they also may be effective up to 5 days after sex. Overall, EC is 95% effective when taken within 5 days after intercourse.

What is the difference between EC and abortion?

EC and abortion are not the same thing. Abortion terminates an existing pregnancy. EC prevents conception by impeding ovulation or implantation after sexual intercourse. EC will not end or harm an existing embryo and therefore cannot be used to induce abortion. Susan Wood, a professor at George Washington University, explains: "These products [EC pills] are not abortifacients. . . . And their only connection to abortion is that they can prevent the need for one" (Rovner, 2013).

Where can I purchase EC?

The Paragard® IUD is not available over the counter. It must be prescribed by and inserted by a physician. Similarly, the EC pill Ella® is only available via prescription. As of 2019, however, progestin, sometimes called the "morning-after pill," is available over the counter at most drugstores and pharmacies in the United States to people of any age, gender, or circumstance. The price of a copper IUD varies widely depending on an individual's health-care plan. Ella® usually costs $50–$70. Over the counter progestin pills cost anywhere from $20 to $50.

How old do I have to be to purchase EC?

In 2012, women over the age of 17 were legally permitted to purchase the progestin EC pill over the counter. However, as of 2019, people of any age and gender may purchase progestin-based EC pills over the counter.

What are the benefits of dual protection?

Dual protection is defined as a method of birth control that also protects against STIs. Unfortunately, the most effective methods of contraception (sterilization and LARC methods) do not also prevent the transmission of STIs. Other forms of birth control, however, such as the male condom or female condom, when used correctly and consistently, are effective in preventing both pregnancy and STIs. Using condoms, then, can be beneficial because they provide dual protection. Dual protection can also be achieved by using a highly effective method of contraception and a male or female condom. In our research, many women used dual protection. According to one woman, "I guess I always thought that you should be using condoms and the pill, just as a rule, just because that is the safest thing I can think of, and the most convenient."

A brief history of birth control

The notion that before the modern age, women had no control over their fertility and, as a result, were subject to endless unwanted pregnancies is a myth. There is no particular historical moment when birth control was invented. In fact, people have tried to control reproduction since the beginning of human existence. For most people with limited resources, having too many children was a burden, and having children too close together also increased the danger of complications during childbirth. Historians claim that low birth rates despite early age at marriage in different premodern times and places, such as parts of the Roman Empire and medieval Italian cities, prove that these populations deliberately controlled fertility through what John M. Riddle calls "human intervention" (Riddle, 1992, p. 1). The methods used by premodern populations (discussed later in this chapter) varied, and their success rates did as well. It is important to note that, depending on the time and place, factors including socioeconomic status, marital status, race or ethnicity, ability, religion, and more could affect one's ability to control fertility as well as access to different methods of birth control. Table 2.1 provides a brief summary of the history of birth control.

How and why have fertility rates and demographic trends changed over time?

While the history of birth control is one of continuity—a story of people across time and space trying to control pregnancy and birth—it is also a narrative of significant transformations.

Table 2.1 A Brief Chronology of Birth Control

Time	Event
2000 BCE	In Egypt, the Kahun Gynecological Papyrus describes how to use honey and crocodile dung as spermicides and cervical plugs.
1600s CE	Barrier methods, including condoms made of animal intestines, begin to be used in some parts of Europe mostly for disease prevention.
1800s CE	
1839	Charles Goodyear invents the technology to vulcanize rubber and manufactures rubber condoms, intrauterine devices, and diaphragms.
1842	The diaphragm is invented in Germany.
1873	The US Congress passes the Comstock Act, which makes it a federal offense to distribute contraceptives through the postal service or across state lines.
1895	The first patent for an intrauterine contraceptive device (IUD) is issued.
1900s CE	
1906	The first spermicidal jelly, Patentex, is available in the United States.
1907	The first forced sterilization law in the United States is passed in Indiana.
1914	Margaret Sanger coins the term "birth control" in the June 1914 issue of *The Woman Rebel*.
1916	Margaret Sanger is arrested for opening the first U.S. birth control clinic in Brooklyn, New York.
1918	The Crane decision is the first legal ruling allowing birth control to be used for therapeutic purposes.

Table 2.1   Continued

Time	Event
1920s CE	
1921	Margaret Sanger establishes the American Birth Control League, the antecedent of the Planned Parenthood Federation of America.
1923	Following the Crane decision, Margaret Sanger opens the first legal birth control clinic in the United States to provide contraceptives for medical purposes.
1936	In *U.S. vs. One Package*, the court rules that physicians can receive contraception via the mail unless prohibited by a specific local law.
1940s CE	
1941	Chemist Russell Marker uses Mexican wild yams known as *cabeza de negro* to make synthetic progesterone, which will become the basis for hormonal contraception.
1944	Gregory Pincus founds a small, private laboratory in Shrewsbury, Massachusetts, to pursue research on hormonal contraception.
1946–1954	The baby boom occurs in the United States.
1950s CE	
1950	The Planned Parenthood Federation of America operates 200 birth control clinics. Anti–birth control laws on the books in 30 states still prohibit or restrict counseling and sale of contraception.
1954	Gregory Pincus and John Rock, MD, begin the first human trials of hormonal contraception. The regimen still in use today is established where progesterone is administered for only 21 days, followed by a 7-day break initiating withdrawal bleeding to mimic menstruation, which allows oral contraception to be seen as a "natural" process.
1956	Rock and Pincus launch the first large-scale human clinical trials for oral contraception in San Juan, Puerto Rico.
1957	The U.S. Food and Drug Administration (FDA) approves the use of Enovid for the treatment of severe menstrual disorders and requires the drug label to carry the warning that Enovid will suppress ovulation.

(*continued*)

Table 2.1   Continued

Time	Event
1960s CE	
1960	FDA approves Searle's Enovid as a "birth control pill."
1965	The U.S. Supreme Court in *Griswold v. Connecticut* strikes down the Connecticut law prohibiting the use of birth control as a violation of a couple's right to privacy. More than 6 million American women use the pill as their main form of contraception.
1968	Pope Paul VI publishes *Humanae Vitae*, which affirms the Catholic Church's opposition to all forms of "artificial" birth control.
1969	Women around the world begin using the contraceptive shot/injection.
1970s CE	
1970	The first patent for the development of the vaginal contraception ring is issued; Title X of the Public Service Act provides funding for family planning services for low-income women.
1972	The U.S. Supreme Court overturns Massachusetts law prohibiting the sale of contraceptives to unmarried women.
1973	The FDA rejects application for the contraception shot/injection, despite committee's recommendation for approval.
1980s CE	The FDA reports that 10.7 million American women use oral hormonal contraception. New versions of low-dosage oral contraceptives are introduced.
1990s	
1990	The FDA approves the first contraception implant/rod.
1992	The FDA approves the contraception shot/injection (Depo-Provera®).
1993	The *Economist* names the birth control pill one of the "Seven Wonders of the Modern World."
2000s CE	
2001	The FDA approves the first vaginal contraception ring (NuvaRing®) and the first transdermal contraception patch (Ortho Evra®) for use by women in the United States.
2012	In a poll, 90% of Americans declare their support for birth control.
2012	The Affordable Care Act includes a "contraceptive mandate" requiring most American employers to offer cost-free birth control.

Table 2.1 Continued

Time	Event
2014	In *Burwell vs. Hobby Lobby*, the Supreme Court decides that some employers may opt out of the Affordable Care Act's contraceptive mandate if birth control conflicts with their religious beliefs.
2018	The FDA removes Essure from the American market.
2019	Current research focuses on extended cycle vaginal birth control rings, transdermal contraception and antimicrobial sprays and gel, and male hormonal contraception, among others.
2019	The Trump administration's "domestic gag rule" prohibits Title X-funded organizations from providing abortion services or abortion referrals.

This timeline is based on (Sundstrom, 2015) and constructed through review of a variety of other sources (Collins, 2009; Foley, 1999; Tone, 2001; Upadhyay, 2005).

There are a few distinct eras of change that are particularly noteworthy. At the beginning of the modern era (1800s–1900s) in the West (here, meaning western Europe and the United States), notable changes in fertility control occurred. The overall pattern here is one of decreasing fertility. Since approximately 1800, "every successfully developing country experienced a fertility transition: starting at initially high levels, fertility rates went down towards a low plateau, oftentimes below replacement level" (Strulik & Vollmer, 2015, p. 32). The changes involving declining fertility rates sometimes are called "fertility transitions" or even "contraceptive revolutions" (McLaren, 1992, p. 2). Most European countries, alongside the United States, began to see the effects of these declining fertility rates in the mid-to-late 1800s. In the nineteenth-century United States, White women's birth rates declined by 50%—from 7.04 at the beginning of the century to 3.56 by the end of the century (Smith, 1973, p. 43). It is clear that these shifting rates were the effect of direct human intervention, meaning family planning. The reasons for the timing

of the nineteenth-century fertility transition remain somewhat obscure, although historians have linked declining fertility to a number of factors including industrialization and
falling mortality rates at the time.

Within the overall trend of decreasing fertility in the United
States since the 1800s, we also witness some bursts of increased
fertility. The most well-known of these is the post–World War
II baby boom, which occurred from 1946 to 1964. Americans
born during these years are known as "baby boomers." After
the end of World War II in 1945, American birth rates increased
rapidly and continued to do so for decades. For every 1,000
women of childbearing age, there was a birth rate of 122.7 in
1957 (the peak of the "boom"), compared to 75.8 births per
1,000 women in 1936. Historians don't necessarily agree on the
reasons for this increase, but most would argue that people
desired to create families and "normal" lives after the destruction of war as well as the Great Depression that preceded it in
the 1930s. In addition, the war may have delayed the ability
of some younger people to marry and start families, so the
baby boom may have been an attempt to "catch up" by some
people. Moreover, a postwar economic boom made it financially possible for some Americans to marry young and have
more children.

American fertility rates declined once more, however, in the
late 1960s and early 1970s, in part because of modern forms
of contraception (discussed later in this chapter). Again, the
overall story of fertility rates in the modern era in the United
States is one of decline. This is not necessarily a global pattern,
however. After 1950, and continuing to today, the developed
world and the developing world diverged in terms of fertility
rates. While the developed world, including the United States,
began to adopt a low-fertility model, high fertility rates persisted in parts of the developing world.

It is important to note that not all historical eras of significance in the United States were associated with marked

fertility transitions or the entire population. The era of slavery, for example, often ignored in histories of birth control, was vitally important. In the American South before 1865, when the system of slavery reigned, reproduction was at the center of concern. Slave owners encouraged fertility among enslaved women because the system could only survive with the birth of enslaved children and thus the creation of more "workers." In the early nineteenth century, slave owners and doctors teamed up to monitor the fertility of enslaved women and attempt to increase their birth rates. Within this particular historical context, "black women's reproductive roles became politically, as well as economically, decisive" (Schwartz, 2006, p. 15), and enslaved women's fertility was enforced by oppression and violence. Even during this time, however, enslaved women attempted to control fertility via birth control and abortion. Historians including Jennifer Morgan (2004) have asserted that these efforts amounted to a form of resistance to slavery. The significance of both the attempted control of the reproductive capacities of enslaved women and their resistance to this is evident when we recognize that such patterns persisted long after the emancipation of African Americans in the United States (see the following discussion of reproductive coercion). The example of enslaved women and birth control also reminds us that reproduction, fertility, and contraception always intersect with economic and political realities and that they have different meanings across time and space.

What were historical methods of birth control?

Historical methods of birth control are as varied as human societies themselves. Before modern forms of contraception were invented in the 1800s and 1900s, people employed various tactics to control fertility. Some were similar to methods we have today: behavioral modification methods, abstinence, and barrier methods all appear to have been common. Other methods, which we would not consider birth control or contraception today, also were used to control fertility. Infanticide is one of these, although it is impossible to produce accurate statistics. In premodern societies in particular, infanticide or the killing of an infant likely was common and, depending on the time and place, considered to be less morally offensive than it is now. Infanticide could occur in several ways. A newly born infant could be smothered, strangled, or otherwise killed deliberately. Other techniques, however, involved the abandonment or exposure of infants, who then might die from natural causes or be taken away by animals. Of course, some of these children may have been found by, or even adopted by, other people.

Not all people without modern forms of contraception resorted to infanticide, however. Written records describing contraception have been around for centuries. Some of the first documented accounts of contraceptives were produced in ancient Egypt. The Kahun Gynecological Papyrus, written in approximately 2000 BCE, described how to use substances including honey and crocodile dung—mixed and inserted into the vagina before penetrative sex—as spermicides and cervical plugs. The ancient Greeks and Romans also had much to say about fertility control. Plato wrote of the "many devices" that women could use to prevent pregnancy, and douching after intercourse appears to have been popular in ancient Rome (Riddle, 1997).

In addition, before the modern era, periodic abstinence likely was common and utilized to prevent unwanted births. Accounts from Europe in the 1600s detail strategies including sleeping in separate beds and having children sleeping in the bed with a couple to prevent or avoid intercourse. In the seventeenth century, a French aristocrat wrote to her daughter, who had birthed three children quickly after marriage, "I beg you, my love, do not trust the two beds; it is a subject of temptation.

Have someone sleep in your room." Later she wrote, "If [your husband] falls into temptation, don't believe he loves you! Continue this nice custom of sleeping separately, and restore yourself" (Wheaton, 1980, p. 141).

Although we recognize today that coitus interruptus or withdrawal before ejaculation is not one of the most reliable forms of birth control, options in the past were limited, and in all premodern societies, this has been documented as a popular way to try to limit births. Evidence from Renaissance Italy is sinister but also telling. In a 1457 criminal court case involving an incest charge, the defendant explicitly admitted to the court that when he had sexual intercourse with his daughter, "He . . . coming together with her when he came to the moment of emitting sperm, withdrew his member and ejected semen between the thighs of the said Antonia because he said that he did not wish to impregnate her" (Ruggiero, 1989, p. 42).

Barrier methods, although less effective than the ones we have today, also predominated. Prophylactics or condoms made from animal intestines were available as early as the 16th century in Europe. Condoms initially were used mainly to protect against diseases, especially by men having sex with prostitutes. In an age in which syphilis had become a major scourge in Europe, the condom came to be associated with it and thus was not considered respectable or suitable for married couples for centuries to come. Early condoms were made of pig intestines, tied at the base of the penis, and were washable and reusable. Condoms, however, remained relatively expensive until the twentieth century. In Europe and the United States, by the nineteenth century the language describing condoms was vast and varied. Some called them "baudruches, French letters, safes, armour, and machines. The French referred to condoms as redingotes Anglaises (English riding coats) and capotes Anglaises (English capes)" ("19th Century Artifacts," n.d.).

Other barrier methods used to block the cervix were known as well. A precursor to the diaphragm or cervical cap, the pessary is a "substance or device inserted into the vagina that blocks, repels, or otherwise neutralizes sperm" (Tone, 2001, p. 13). Before the vulcanization of rubber, pessaries or cervical plugs could be constructed out of natural substances, including cotton, wax, coins, stones, or sea sponges. Lemons cut in half allegedly were common as well. Natural substances applied to the genitals to be used as spermicides also proliferated in U.S. history. Vaginal suppositories containing quinine, for example, were known in early America. Although we often think of IUDs as modern forms of birth control, they have been used for centuries. According to Andrea Tone, "Arabs and Turks used hollow tubes to insert small stones into the uteri of camels before long desert trips. This technique was likely used to inhibit human procreation at about the same time" (Tone, 2001, p. 59).

Another popular method used across time and space was douching. Douching describes a process when a woman washes, cleans, or flushes out the vagina with a liquid. Women douched after intercourse with a substance such as vinegar to kill or damage sperm and thus prevent conception. This practice persisted across centuries and across continents. By the 1800s in the United States, it had become a well-known method of birth control. Douching, in fact, has been called "the first modern method" of American birth control, and in 1832, it was even mentioned in a book written by a physician, Charles Knowlton, who wrote that a way of preventing conception was by "syringing the vagina immediately after connection with a solution of sulphate of zinc, of alum, pearl-ash, or any salt that acts chemically on the semen" (Knowlton, 1832).

Aside from coitus interruptus, perhaps the most common premodern form of birth control that lasted into the modern era was the consuming of potions, herbs, or tonics to either prevent conception or induce miscarriage. These methods were constant, in fact, across centuries and still were used in the early twentieth century in the United States. In sixteenth- and seventeenth-century England and later in colonial America, these substances were commonly known as "physick," and some potions were written down in what were called "receipt," or recipe, books. Examples of contraceptive recipes exist from Asia to Europe. In 1597, for example, an Englishman, William Langham (1597), wrote: "The flowers of a Sallow or Willow, maketh cold all heat of carnal lust and causeth barrenness. Poplar tree bark, he also claimed, made women barren "if drunk with the kidney of a mule." Naturally occurring substances used as physick, which were believed to have contraceptive characteristics, included myrrh, juniper, and pennyroyal.

People's views of contraception in the past sometimes were different from our own views. More specifically, before the twentieth century, most people did not draw sharp lines between contraception and abortion. Preventing a birth and inducing a miscarriage during an early stage of pregnancy were considered to be similar acts that produced the same effect. Before accurate pregnancy tests and modern imaging, the signs of pregnancy were ambiguous. Menstruation could stop for several reasons, including malnutrition. Most women, therefore, were not certain that they were pregnant until they felt the fetus "quickening" or moving/fluttering within the womb. This usually occurs around the fourth or fifth month of a pregnancy. Therefore, in most people's minds, herbal tonics and potions that were consumed early in a pregnancy to restore menstruation (what we would call abortion-causing agents, emmenagogues, or abortifacients) were thought of as the same as substances designed to prevent conception. People in the eighteenth and nineteenth centuries conflated abortion-causing substances and substances designed to prevent conception. Views that abortion is fundamentally different from contraception, or even that abortion is the destruction of a potentially viable fetus or embryo, are recent. By the twentieth century, scientists discovered the differences between contraception and abortion. While contraception prevents fertilization, abortion eliminates a fertilized egg. So today, we understand that substances that cause abortion (abortifacients) are distinct from contraceptive substances such as the pill or EC methods such as the morning-after pill. These distinctions, however, were not shared by our ancestors. Again, until recently, there was no clear distinction or moral difference between consuming substances for both contraception and abortion.

When Europeans colonized the Americas, physick, including contraceptives and emmenagogues, also crossed the Atlantic. Londa Schiebinger's (2007) work has shown that, across the eighteenth-century Atlantic World, women used plants and herbs to bring on uterine contractions and thus end pregnancies. In 1742, in Pomfret, Connecticut, a man was brought to court on murder charges after he gave an unspecified abortifacient, in drug form, to his young lover. After miscarrying, the woman died. Native Americans also had their own physick. Quinine, for example, native to the Americas, was and still is a substance used to bring on uterine contractions, whether to hasten labor and birth or induce a miscarriage. By the eighteenth century in the United States, enslaved peoples used cotton root, which already was well known in parts of Africa as an abortifacient. According to Laurie Wilkie (2013),

> in southern African-American oral histories, senna and castor oil are important as abortifacients and to aid contractions during childbirth. Other products used reported during the period of enslavement include cotton seed, cedar berries, camphor, asafetida, quinine, rust, juniper, snakeroot, Jamaican ginger and turpentine. (p. 275)

In our interviews conducted in 2016, African American women in South Carolina reported that many of these traditional methods of contraception and abortion passed down orally across the generations. When asked how women tried to control their fertility before contraception and abortion were readily available, an interviewee answered, "Well, I think there were ways. I think that in our [African American] community, even in Charleston, there were certain . . . slave women eating certain herbs when they were being raped against their will." Another woman recalled her mother's advice in the 1960s: "Now I remember when I was in high school my mother saying to me, 'If you ever feel like you're pregnant, come to me and I will give you some pills. Some quinine.' " One interviewee recalled watching her family members force an approximately 14-year-old girl to sit at the table and drink a mixture of turpentine, vinegar, and water. She told us that "a few days later [the girl] did abort her baby." Yet another interviewee remembered women obtaining oral abortifacients through traditional healers such as "root doctors," or nonprescription medicines that they heard would procure miscarriages:

> Women would go to . . . these root doctors, as they were called, to get potions to end pregnancies. Women would also O.D. on laxatives. That's right. Not just get everything out, but get your system geared up so the only thing that's left is something in your uterus. Body's still gonna constrict because it's there.

It is important to recognize, then, that well into the twentieth century, despite the increased availability of more "modern" forms of birth control, traditions persisted.

When were modern methods of birth control invented?

The Centers for Disease Control and Prevention recognizes modern contraception as one of the most important public health developments of the twentieth century. Modern methods of birth control, including products made from rubber and plastic as well as hormonal contraceptive pills and devices, began to appear in the nineteenth and twentieth centuries, although their origins came from earlier centuries.

Some of the most significant inventions in birth control history were tied to the 1839 actions of Charles Goodyear. Goodyear was an American inventor who discovered how to vulcanize or chemically alter rubber by heating it. Once rubber was able to be vulcanized, it transformed the manufacture and marketing of contraceptives including condoms and diaphragms. Late nineteenth-century condoms that were made of rubber were washable and reusable; it was not until the 1930s and 1940s that latex rubber condoms, including those manufactured under the brand Trojan®, became inexpensive, disposable, and relatively common. Part of the reason for this was because of the two world wars. Fears that soldiers, traveling overseas and presumably having sex with prostitutes, would contract and spread what was called venereal disease led the U.S. government to encourage soldiers to use condoms, which made many men familiar with them; these men would continue to utilize condoms after the wars. Condom use in the United States, in fact, peaked in the 1940s and 1950s but began to decline in the 1960s and 1970s after the birth control pill became more popular (Lieberman, 2017). The female condom was not perfected and available for use in the United States until the 1980s.

The first modern diaphragm was also tied to the nineteenth century. Invented in 1842 in Germany, it grew steadily in popularity across Europe and the United States. U.S. doctor Edward Bliss Foote, in the 1860s and 1870s, developed what he called a "womb veil" likely made simply of rubber-covered wire. The diaphragm, often used in conjunction with spermicidal jelly, became the most used form of contraception by the 1930s. Although the diaphragm needed to be fitted by a physician, many women at the time preferred the diaphragm to condoms because using it did not require male cooperation.

Modern cervical caps and sponges, although less popular than diaphragms, also increased in use in the early to mid-twentieth century. In 1906, the first modern spermicidal jelly, called Patentex, became available for purchase in the United States.

Also in the first decade of the twentieth century, the first commercially available IUD was marketed. Before this, however, in the late 1800s, a plethora of IUDs were available, and American doctors actively worked to create marketable devices. Because IUDs could be used not just for contraception but also to control menstrual bleeding as well as "for a wide range of gynecological disorders," they were difficult to regulate, even under the Comstock Act (Tone, 2001, p. 59). Hormonal IUDs were not available until the 1960s, after the development of synthetic hormones (discussed later in this chapter). In 1968, the FDA approved IUDs as a form of birth control.

Although douching is certainly not a "modern" form of birth control, by the early 1900s, it began to be marketed and distributed in modern ways. Even when it became clear, by the early twentieth century, that douching likely was not an effective method of preventing conception, the practice continued and, in fact, may have even expanded because of the advent of mass media. In the early twentieth-century United States, advertisements for douching kits appeared in numerous newspapers and magazines, and thousands of women purchased such kits either at local pharmacies or via mail order catalogues. Advertisers often referred to "feminine hygiene" rather than "douching," and this term, although understood by people at the time to reference fertility control, reflected the new twentieth-century focus on cleanliness and hygiene that would intersect with contraceptive technology (Ferranti, 2009, p. 599). Douching with Lysol was something, according to the mass media, that women could do for both cleanliness and contraception. In 1933, for example, the popular *McCall's* magazine published the following advertisement:

> The most frequent eternal triangle:
> A HUSBAND . . . A WIFE . . . and her fears
> Fewer marriages would flounder around in a maze of misunderstanding and unhappiness if more wives knew and practiced regular marriage hygiene. Without it, some minor physical irregularity plants in a woman's mind the fear of a major crisis. Let so devastating a fear recur again and again, and the most gracious wife turns into a nerve-ridden, irritable travesty of herself, (Tone, 1997, p. 211)

The involvement of mass production and mass marketing in birth control that was evident in the case of douching would create a precedent for the future and would particularly affect birth control pill consumption.

Advances in hormonal contraception, which would lead to the invention of the birth control pill, originated with scientific developments related to hormone research in the 1940s and 1950s. In the 1940s, Russell Earl Marker produced synthetic progesterone made from Mexican yams. The creation of artificial hormones paved the way for modern hormonal forms of birth control. Throughout the 1950s, scientists continued attempts to produce synthetic hormones that would help regulate the female reproductive system. The American company Searle sponsored the research of Gregory Pincus, who, in 1957, created Enovid, a pill made up of synthetic estrogen and progesterone. The FDA approved Enovid to treat severe menstrual disorders, and in 1960, it was approved in the United States for consumption as a contraceptive. Hormonal contraception, now on the map, would transform birth control in the ensuing years. By 1965, more than six million American women used the pill as their main form of contraception.

In 1962, a freelance writer named Gloria Steinem published an article in *Esquire* in which she predicted that the pill would create a whole new generation of young women who would be "free to take sex, education, work, and even marriage when and how they like." Activists at the time argued that the pill was a revolutionary invention for women. They claimed that it uniquely empowered women to manage their own fertility. Some methods, notably condoms, require male cooperation to be successful. Using a pessary or diaphragm requires that couples pause for a moment or two before actual intercourse to insert the device. Now, however, by the 1960s, women could manage their own fertility, on their own, with no one else's assistance or even knowledge. This allowed many women to separate sex from reproduction. The pill, in fact, helped create the sexual revolution and fueled a new feminist movement. Over time, the pill also affected women's public participation. For example, it became harder in the 1960s for employers to deny women access to jobs on the grounds that their inevitable pregnancies would cause them to leave.

The statistics of OCP use in the United States since 1960 are staggering. By 1961, two million American women were taking the pill regularly. In 1966, that figure reached six million, and a year later, in 1967, *Time* magazine was touting the pill as revolutionary. By 1990, 80% of American women born since the end of World War II had been on the pill at some point in their lives. In 1993, *The Economist* even named the pill one of the "Seven Wonders of the Modern World." Today, the pill is a part of the everyday lives of 10.5 million American women.

LARC methods of birth control, recommended today as particularly effective, also trace their history to the early to midtwentieth century. As mentioned earlier, forms of IUDs were used by thousands of American women from the 1850s to 1950s. By the late 1960s, copper and plastic IUDs were mass manufactured and marketed. However, fears after the controversies surrounding the Dalkon Shield in the early 1970s (see Chapter 1 of this volume) curbed the IUD's popularity and growth. The ParaGard® copper IUD made its appearance on the American market in the late 1980s, and the hormonal IUD (Mirena®) in the early 2000s. Skyla®, Liletta®, and Kyleena® were approved in quick succession over a decade later beginning in 2013.

The first hormonal implant, Norplant, was marketed to American women in 1991. Within three years, over a million women were using it as their primary method of contraception. Its use declined in the following years, however, as women began to complain about side effects and a lack of training of physicians on how to properly insert and remove it. It was not until 2006 that a new implant, Nexplanon®, would make inroads in the United States.

How have laws about birth control changed over time?

While humans have always attempted to control fertility, the contexts in which they do so have changed. Most laws legislating birth control have focused on contraceptive methods rather than abstinence or behavior modification methods. In 1873, most forms of contraception became illegal in the United States under the Comstock Act. This legislation targeted "obscene," "lewd," lascivious," "immoral," or "indecent" literature, including birth control. Punishments for breaking the new law included fines and possible imprisonment. The Comstock Act targeted in particular publications about contraception that were transmitted through the U.S. mail. It did not, however, criminalize other forms of birth control that did not intersect with financial markets. "Traditional" methods including natural family planning and abstinence, for example, remained permissible, accepted, and, indeed, almost impossible to detect. Tone (2001) argues that criminalization of contraception was linked to its growing "commercial visibility"; this theory, she claims, helps explain why more "traditional" methods were overlooked completely (p. 13). By the late nineteenth century, in fact, magazines and newspapers were flooded with advertisements for not only new rubber sheaths and diaphragms but also for "female pills" and "menstrual regulators" that had abortifacient properties. At a time when the first wave of feminist activism was beginning, industrialization and urbanization had transformed "traditional" family life, and Americans became obsessed with crime and immorality, the regulation of contraception was part and parcel of a new moral movement to reform society and culture and prevent degeneration.

What some called reform, however, others experienced as regulation. By the early twentieth century, opponents of censorship and advocates for birth control access and education began to express themselves more openly. Emma Goldman, a Jewish nurse-midwife and anarchist, was one of the first people in the United States to publicly advocate for the decriminalization of birth control. "She began to take direct action in the 1910s, smuggling contraceptive devices into the United States, lecturing frequently on 'the right of the child not to be born' and demanding that women's bodies be freed from the coercion of the government" ("Women of Valor," n.d.). In fact, it was Goldman who inspired and counseled Margaret Sanger, the woman often considered to be the pioneer of birth control in the United States.

Sanger, creator of the Planned Parenthood Federation of America, became a vehement advocate for birth control. In 1919, she argued:

We maintain that a woman possessing an adequate knowledge of her reproductive functions is the best judge of the time and conditions under which her child should be brought into this world. We further maintain that it is her right, regardless of all other considerations, to determine whether she shall bear children or not, and how many children she shall bear if she chooses to become a mother. To this end we insist that information in regard to scientific contraceptives be made open to all.

This, one of the first clearly articulated and one of the most commonly cited, twentieth-century defenses of women's rights to birth control, would pave the way for future debates on contraception for decades to come. In 1936, Sanger's work facilitated the federal court ruling, *United States vs. One Package of Japanese Pessaries*, which helped to overturn the Comstock Act. This 1936 decision declared that doctors should be able to provide contraceptives to their patients free from government regulation or interference. Therefore, theoretically at least, contraception, when prescribed by a physician, was decriminalized in the 1930s.

Still, laws in at least 30 U.S. states continued to regulate or outlaw contraception. By the 1960s, the coming of age of a new postwar generation (the baby boomers) facilitated new cultural and political movements that would, in turn, affect attitudes toward, and laws about, contraception. Individual states controlled people's legal access to contraception until 1965, when the Supreme Court, in *Griswold vs. Connecticut*, ruled that married couples had the right to use birth control because the Constitution protected their right to privacy. Even after 1965, however, 26 states still outlawed birth control for unmarried women. This changed in 1972, when a legal case from Massachusetts made its way to the Supreme Court. In this case, the law, which criminalized contraceptive use for unmarried people, was deemed unconstitutional. As of the 1970s, then, most Americans, whatever their marital status, could use contraceptives legally.

Legal contexts are important, but they don't always tell us about practices or popular attitudes. While some laws in history outlawed contraception, that did not mean that contraceptive use stopped. Enforcement of laws could be sporadic, and many people also defied the law and continued to use contraceptive devices. Similarly, suppliers of contraceptive products did not stop making these items and substances. After the Comstock Act, some used "creative relabeling" to continue to not only produce but also advertise their products. Rather than calling condoms "birth control," for example, manufacturers marketed them as "protection" (Tone, 2001, p. 30). These strategies allowed companies and consumers to continue to sell and buy contraceptives through a coded language that was understood by all but usually not specific enough to be subject to prosecution. Similarly, physicians could prescribe forms of contraception for use other than birth control; this allowed women to, in the words of one of our interviewees, work with doctors to "beat the system." This woman, who was in her 60s when interviewed in 2016, said that she and her friends in the 1960s got the birth control pill by using clever language: "Or if you took birth control pills, it wasn't because you were sexually active, it was because they were to regulate your period."

What is the history of reproductive coercion related to birth control?

The history of birth control in the United States, unfortunately, involves coercive and violent practices. Across centuries, women of color, persons with disabilities, incarcerated women, and immigrants have been the targets of reproductive violence and coercion, including forced childbirth, forced sterilization, or sterilization without consent. Other less direct attempts at coercion, including encouraging particular methods of birth control or not presenting a range of options or adequate and correct information, affect primarily women of low socioeconomic status, young women, women with disabilities, and women of color. Today, these populations are more likely to be encouraged to use permanent or long-acting methods of contraception, including sterilization, than are other women.

In the United States, women of color have been the most common victims of reproductive coercion. In the era of slavery, White slaveowners manipulated the bodies of enslaved women for their own monetary benefit. Slaveholders forced enslaved people into heterosexual partnerships to encourage reproduction. When enslaved women had children, those children automatically became the legal property of the slaveowner. Reproduction thus was key to the entire system of slavery. The birth of an infant to an enslaved mother provided, over time, additional free labor to the slaveowners. At times, owners would use the so-called stud system and impregnate several different women with one enslaved man who was thought to be particularly virile and suited to hard physical labor. This reproductive control was a form of violence against African American women's bodies. It was done not only to maximize the economic gains of the slaveowners but also to solidify the slaveowner's control of the bodies of the enslaved. After emancipation, the violence enacted on African American women's bodies continued, and in the twentieth century, other women of color, as well as immigrants, single mothers, poor women, and women with disabilities, also suffered.

Forced sterilization has a particularly damaging legacy in the United States. The first law in the United States that allowed forced sterilization came into effect in Indiana in 1907. This law stated:

> It shall be compulsory for each and every institution in the state, entrusted with the care of confirmed criminals, idiots, rapists and imbeciles, to appoint upon its staff, in addition to the regular institutional physician, two skilled surgeons of recognized ability, whose duty it shall be, in conjunction with the chief physician of the institution, to examine the mental and physical condition of such inmates as are recommended by the institutional physician and board of managers. If, in the judgment of this committee of experts and the board of managers, procreation is inadvisable and there is no probability of improvement of the mental condition of the inmate, it shall be lawful for the surgeons to perform such operation for the prevention of procreation as shall be decided safest and most effective.

At the time, the eugenics movement, which was enormously popular in the United States, led to attempts to control the reproduction of "undesirable" women. Eugenics is an ideology that advocates for selective breeding—restricting the ability of some people to reproduce while encouraging reproduction in other groups of people.

Across 30 states, similar laws persisted until the 1970s. From the 1940s to the 1970s, North Carolina sterilized over 7,000 women and girls without their consent. Historians such as Johanna Schoen have highlighted the racist, sexist, and classist properties of sterilization policies throughout twentieth-century America (Schoen, 2005). As Schoen (2005) writes,

> sexual behavior, race, and class background constituted major factors in the identification of the so-called feebleminded. A concern with sexual behavior led social workers to focus on those whose deviation from the desired norm was particularly obvious and disturbing: sexually active single women. Eighty-five percent of those sterilized in North Carolina were women, and half of them were single and had given birth to one or more children outside of marriage. (p. 76)

Forced sterilization continued as late as the 1970s in Latina, African American, and Native American communities. In 1973 Alabama, two African American girls aged 12 and 14 were sterilized without their or their parents' consent. Physicians in this case told the girls' mother that they were receiving a contraceptive injection, which she consented to. The girls then, however, were sterilized (Gold, 2014; Meier, Sundstrom, & DeMaria, 2015). Native American women endured forced sterilization and abortion in Indian Health Service clinics throughout most of the twentieth century. In 1978, a court case involving Mexican-American women publicized the phenomenon of forced sterilization. The case revealed that 10 Mexican

American women had been forcibly sterilized from 1971 and 1974 (Meier et al., 2015). In California, between 2006 and 2010, over one hundred incarcerated women were sterilized without their informed consent.

Today, contraceptive coercion remains problematic. Women of color, single mothers, and poor women are encouraged to pursue LARC methods or sterilization more than other women. Women we interviewed, particularly African American women, were conscious of the damaging history of reproductive coercion in the United States and linked it clearly to their concerns about birth control today. One woman stated: "I personally think they [doctors] just want more Black women to use the IUD so they will not have babies." Discussing LARC methods, another said, "I don't know whether I should be offended by this a little bit because I feel like you're offering me an IUD not because it would be helpful to me but because you don't want me to have babies." And a third expressed her thoughts about the government's role in reproductive coercion, past and present:

If you go back and you look at all the per capita income and everything of 30 to 40 years ago down in [rural areas], the uneducated, whether you were White and uneducated, or Black and uneducated. There was always this fear that the government was coming in and the government was giving you something that would stop you from having children, and the idea of taking birth control, the fear was, okay, I can control having a baby and not having a baby, but what happens if I want to have a baby?

3

HOW DO WE KNOW IF BIRTH CONTROL IS SAFE?

Hormonal contraceptive options are among the most well-studied medicines available today. Decades of research and experience show that they are safe. For more than 50 years, millions of women have taken "the pill" safely. Although hormonal birth control is safe for almost all women, any medicine has side effects (positive and negative) and risks. There are more low dose hormonal contraceptive options today that lower the risk of serious side effects. In addition, hormonal contraception offers numerous health benefits to women, including lowering the risk of certain types of cancer.

In this chapter, we organize the available research and evidence on the safety of birth control. Sources include the World Health Organization, the Centers for Disease Control and Prevention, the American College of Obstetricians and Gynecologists (ACOG), and the leading medical text, *Contraceptive Technology* (Hatcher et al., 2018) among others.

The most reliable scientific evidence comes from well-designed experiments. Of these experiments, *randomized controlled trials* are the gold standard: they feature an experimental group and a control group, with the former receiving the experimental therapy and the latter receiving a placebo. Where such experiments are not possible, or where it is unethical to randomly assign people to receive a certain exposure or placebo, *cohort studies* offer the next most robust form of evidence. A cohort is a group of people; cohort studies follow a group of people prospectively to find out how a certain exposure, such as taking birth control, impacts their health over the long term. This type of study is not able to provide definitive proof of a link between an exposure and a health result (like, say, developing a disease). In fact, cohort studies have a number of limitations, including losing track of participants, which can introduce bias, and the likelihood of missing rare diseases or diseases that take a long time to develop. Still, cohort studies are often cited in news stories, so we must acknowledge their impact on how individuals understand and make decisions about birth control.

We aim to provide the resources and tools for individuals to make an informed decision about birth control. That choice may be to use a specific method of birth control or not to use any method of birth control. There is not one best decision for every person; however, all people who can become pregnant deserve access to the best science and evidence without fear or judgment.

What are the risks of hormonal birth control?

Birth control pills are very safe for most women. Moreover, all methods of birth control are safer than pregnancy and childbirth. The risks associated with hormonal contraception are extremely low for most people. Hormonal methods are associated with a small increased risk of deep vein thrombosis (DVT) or blood clots, stroke, heart attack, and liver tumors. These risks are higher among some people, including those who are older than 35 and smoke more than 15 cigarettes each day. Women who have multiple risk factors or a history of certain health conditions, such as high blood pressure, uncontrolled diabetes, blood clots, stroke, heart attack, liver disease, or migraine headaches with aura, may be at increased risk of health problems from hormonal birth control.

The progestin-only pill, known as the "mini-pill," may re-duce or eliminate some of these risks. The arm implant contains progestin and offers limited risks, including the possibility of an infection from insertion. Depo-Provera®, commonly known as "the shot," contains progestin only. According to ACOG, Depo-Provera® may cause the loss of bone density, which can lead to weaker bones; however, this bone density loss is reversed when the method is stopped. Hormonal intrauterine devices (IUDs) contain progestin. The nonhormonal ParaGard® IUD contains copper. Women with bleeding disorders, an allergy to copper, or Wilson's disease, which causes the body to retain too much copper, should not use ParaGard®. Women with certain sexually transmitted infections or a pelvic infection should not use an IUD. In rare cases, IUDs can cause infections, ovarian cysts, ectopic pregnancy, or puncture the wall of the uterus.

Birth control methods containing estrogen, such as the combined oral contraceptive (COC) pill, the patch, and the vaginal ring, present a slightly increased risk of blood clots. While using these methods, long-distance travel and surgery may increase that risk in the short term. Women are most likely to have a blood clot soon after starting hormonal contraception in the first few months up to the first year. During that time, women should be aware of certain symptoms that may indicate a blood clot. It is helpful to remember ACHES—severe abdominal or stomach pain; severe chest pain, cough, or shortness of breath; severe headache, dizziness, weakness, or numbness; eye problems or speech problems; and/or severe leg pain. These symptoms could indicate a blood clot and require immediate medical attention.

The risk of a blood clot while taking the pill, however, is much lower than the risk of blood clot during pregnancy and childbirth. According to the U.S. Food and Drug Administration (FDA, 2012), the likelihood of developing a blood clot among nonpregnant women who are not using a COC ranges from 1 to 5 out of 10,000 women years (WY). Women years is a measure of person-time, which is an estimate of the population at risk of developing the outcome. Among COC users, the likelihood of developing a blood clot is between 3 and 9 out of 10,000 WY. The risk of a blood clot during pregnancy ranges from 5 to 20 women out of 10,000 WY. Among women in the first 12 weeks postpartum, the likelihood of developing a blood clot ranges from 40 to 65 out of 10,000 WY. According to ACOG, the risk of DVT may be higher among women using the patch or taking birth control pills with a progestin called drospirenone. Still, the risk of DVT is higher during pregnancy and in the postpartum period than when using the patch or taking birth control pills with drospirenone.

What are the risks associated with pregnancy and childbirth?

Media stories about the risk of contraception tend to omit the risks of pregnancy and childbirth. All contraceptive methods are safer than pregnancy and childbirth. Our intent in making this comparison is not to instill fear related to pregnancy and childbirth. Instead, we aim to juxtapose media coverage depicting pregnancy as "natural" with the sensationalized and flawed reports of complications related to contraceptive use. We hope that our analysis helps to disrupt the nature/technology dualism, reconceptualizing health and risk outside of the normative "natural" processes of menstruation, pregnancy, and childbirth (Sundstrom, 2015). In other words, how we define "nature" and "natural" is grounded in our social and cultural understandings of the world. As Haraway (2004) argued, we do not advocate for moving "back" to nature; instead, by sharing scientific evidence, we hope to provide women with the tools to understand and benefit from scientific progress and technology.

In the United States, the maternal mortality rate has doubled over the past 20 years. The Centers for Disease Control and Prevention started collecting national surveillance data about pregnancy-related deaths in 1986. Since that time, reported pregnancy-related deaths have increased from 7.2 deaths per 100,000 live births to 17.2 deaths per 100,000 live births in 2015 (Shah, 2018). To put that into perspective, the United States and Serbia are the only developed nations where maternal mortality rates have increased since 1990. American women today are more likely to die in childbirth than their own mothers. In addition, there are significant racial/ethnic disparities in maternal mortality, with African American women experiencing 3 to 4 times higher maternal morality than White women. Scholars argue that approximately 60% of pregnancy-related deaths are preventable (Solly, 2019). Experts suggest that America is experiencing a maternal mortality crisis.

An analysis of the reasons for the maternal mortality crisis is outside of the scope of this book; however, a reproductive justice framework shows that the issues of contraceptive access and maternal mortality are intertwined, linked through patriarchal systems that perpetuate fear of women's bodies and women's autonomy. The medicalization of pregnancy and childbirth, part of a larger trend toward biomedical approaches to American life, has contributed to this crisis (Davis-Floyd, 2003; Martin, 2001; Pollock, 1999; Wolf, 2011). In 1900, almost all births in the United States took place at home; by 1969 that number was 1% (MacDorman, Mathews, & Declercq, 2012). During this transition, medicalizing childbirth resulted in negative health consequences for women, especially upper-class women, who had the highest maternal mortality rates, likely reflecting their ability to afford a physician instead of a traditional midwife. Rooks (1999) described this phenomenon, stating "whenever and wherever midwifery declined, the incidence of maternal mortality and infant deaths from birth injuries increased" (p. 30). Although the United States is the only developed country without a formal system of midwifery, there have been recent attempts to promote physiological childbirth. In particular, March for Moms is a national multi-stakeholder coalition dedicated to improving the health and wellbeing of mothers in the United States (http://www.

marchformoms.org/). This coalition is led by some of the foremost health-care providers and researchers of maternal health, including Ginger Breedlove, Neel Shah, and Eugene Declercq.

Does hormonal birth control increase the risk of breast cancer?

Studies investigating whether or not hormonal birth control increases the risk of breast cancer remain inconsistent. There is some scientific evidence that using hormonal birth control slightly increases the risk of breast cancer, while other studies find no increased risk. Research shows that women who use oral contraceptives have a decreased risk of benign breast disease compared with nonusers. Among women who have a family history of breast cancer, studies show no link between the use of hormonal birth control and breast cancer risk. There is also a consensus that birth control decreases the risk of other types of cancer, such as ovarian, endometrial, and colorectal cancer. As a result, there is growing evidence that the net effect of using oral contraception is a reduction in the overall risk of cancer. We discuss this evidence on the benefits of hormonal contraception later in this chapter.

One recent study about hormonal contraception and the risk of breast cancer received particular media attention. A 2017 cohort study published in the *New England Journal of Medicine* (Mørch et al., 2017) found that there was a small increased risk of breast cancer among users of hormonal contraception, including pills or IUDs. The authors did not find significant associations among women who had used other types of hormonal contraception, including progestin-only pills, patches, rings, implants, or injectables. Among current and recent users of hormonal contraception, the risk of breast cancer was 13 cases per 100,000 person-years. In other words, using hormonal contraception could result in 1 additional case of breast cancer out of 7,690 women. However, among women younger than 35 years, using hormonal contraception could result in

1 additional case of breast cancer out of 50,000 women. The researchers described important factors that could have impacted the results of the study, including a lack of information on breastfeeding, alcohol consumption, and physical activity, as well as the northern European population, which may limit the generalizability of the findings. As is always the case, cohort studies can describe associations but do not show cause and effect.

Although ACOG urged the media to interpret the small increased risk of breast cancer found in this study in the context of the benefits of hormonal contraception, numerous media outlets sensationalized the limited findings. Headlines such as "Do Hormonal Contraceptives Increase Breast Cancer Risk?" and "The Pill and Cancer: Is There a Link?" appeared in newspapers and websites worldwide. The *New York Times* reported: "Birth Control Pills Still Linked to Breast Cancer, Study Finds" (Rabin, 2017). In the United Kingdom, the *Independent* reported: "Birth Control Pills Have Been Linked to an Increased Risk of Breast Cancer in New Study" (Johnson, 2017). The uncontextualized media attention led ACOG to release a Practice Advisory on Hormonal Contraception and Risk of Breast Cancer. This advisory concluded:

- This recent study showed that women who use hormonal birth control methods may have a small increased risk of breast cancer, but the overall risk of breast cancer in hormonal birth control users remains very low.
- Hormonal birth control is very effective in preventing pregnancy and may lower a women's overall risk of cancer by providing protection against other types of cancer.
- There are nonhormonal methods of birth control that are also good options.
- Women can do things to help lower their risk of breast cancer, like breastfeeding, getting more exercise, and limiting alcohol intake. (ACOG, 2017)

Nancy Keating, a professor of health-care policy and medicine at Harvard Medical School and a physician at Brigham and Women's Hospital, contextualized the study's findings in an article in *Harvard Women's Health Watch*. She said, "So, the increased risk associated with oral contraceptive pills—an extra 13 cancers per 100,000 person-years—is much less than the risk associated with drinking even three to six drinks per week, which is an extra 22 cancers per 100,000 person-years" ("Study Finds Weak Link," 2018).

Findings from another cohort study published in 2017 in the *American Journal of Obstetrics and Gynecology* showed that any increased breast cancer risk in current and recent users of hormonal contraception dissipated within about five years of discontinuing oral contraception (Iversen, Sivasubramaniam, Lee, Fielding, & Hannaford, 2017). Furthermore, the risk of breast cancer did not increase over time in ever uses of hormonal contraception. This study included 44 years of follow up, including 1.3 million women-years of observation, from the Royal College of General Practitioners' Oral Contraception Study, which is the longest running study of oral contraception worldwide. The authors noted that the lack of long-term breast cancer risk mirrors the results of two other cohort studies, including the Nurses' Health Study and the Oxford-Family Planning Association Study.

What are the benefits of hormonal birth control?

In addition to preventing unintended pregnancy, studies show that hormonal contraception offers a net health benefit to users, including treating or preventing the following: anemia, heavy menstrual bleeding (HMB) and cramps, acne, migraines, pelvic inflammatory disease (PID), ovarian cysts, polycystic ovarian syndrome (PCOS), uterine fibroids (myomata), endometriosis, uterine cancer, endometrial cancer, ovarian cancer, and colon cancer.

Can hormonal birth control cause weight gain?

We also want to address some of the common myths about birth control related to weight gain. Women we have talked with have made decisions about contraception based on ideas about weight control. One woman said, "The shot makes you gain weight, the pill makes you gain weight. I don't need to gain any more weight, I'm trying to lose it." Although weight gain may be a side effect of some hormonal contraceptive options, most studies have found no evidence that hormonal contraception causes significant weight gain. Experts suggest that most weight gain while using hormonal contraception is due to water retention, lifestyle changes, or normal aging. In addition, every body is different, so changing to a different hormonal contraceptive option might work better for some women.

Can hormonal birth control cause depression?

In recent years, news media have suggested an association between birth control and depression with headlines such as, "'The Pill' May Raise Depression Risk," "Birth Control and Depression: Understanding the Link," and "Depression and Suicide: The Dark Side of the Birth Control Pill." However, a 2017 double-blind, randomized, placebo-controlled trial found no association between depression and oral contraceptive use (Zethraeus, Dreber, & Ranehill, 2017). This study supports several other studies that found no association between hormonal contraception and depression.

Can hormonal birth control affect fertility later in life?

Another common concern is the impact of hormonal contraception on fertility, especially after long-term use. Women we have talked with have described fears that hormonal contraception will "cover up fertility issues later on." There is no evidence that hormonal contraception negatively impacts fertility; in fact, studies show it may improve future fertility by limiting ovulatory cycles. If you become pregnant while using hormonal contraception, there is no increased risk of birth defects. Many women have reported receiving obsolete advice from their health-care providers, such as, "They said just wait a couple of months just to give your body time to reset." After stopping hormonal contraception, there is no reason to wait to become pregnant. Becoming pregnant immediately does not increase the risk of miscarriage.

Most women will ovulate approximately two weeks after stopping hormonal contraception, which means they can become pregnant before having a period. A recent analysis of 17 studies found that one-year pregnancy rates and outcomes (such as pregnancy complications) among women stopping hormonal contraception were comparable to women using no contraceptive method or barrier methods (Mansour, Gemzell-Danielsson, Inki, & Jensen, 2011). A case-control study found that longer-term use of the oral contraceptive pill (OCP) lowered the risk of Down syndrome in children among women of advanced maternal age and may protect against miscarriage by limiting unnecessary ovulations (Nagy, Gyrffy, Nagy, & Rigó, 2013). Another observational study found that longer use of oral contraception may lower the risk of common fetal trisomies among women of advanced reproductive age (Horányi, Babay, Rigó, Győrffy, & Nagy, 2017). Although more research is needed, experts suggest that limiting the number of ovulations may protect against common fetal trisomies. These studies indicate that hormonal contraception may improve fertility.

Does hormonal contraception treat or prevent heavy menstrual bleeding, premenstrual syndrome, painful periods, and/or acne?

Yes, to all of the above. Conversations on this topic sometimes lead to the question "What constitutes a heavy period?" To this, it is worth heeding the words of Robert A. Hatcher, lead author of the formative book *Contraceptive Technology*, who was once asked at a conference to define HMB. Rather than offering a quantifiable measurement, Hatcher suggested that a woman has HMB "if she says she has heavy menstrual bleeding." In other words, he encouraged health-care providers to listen to women. In the latest edition of *Contraceptive Technology*, Anita Nelson and Lee Shulman (2018) reinforce this approach, noting that a key factor in diagnosing HMB should be the extent to which it disrupts a woman's life.

HMB effects approximately 30% of women. The hormonal IUD (Mirena®) and one oral combined contraceptive (Natazia®) have been approved by the FDA to treat HMB. Doctors may prescribe other oral combined contraceptives off-label to lessen bleeding. The progestin-only pill may control bleeding and the Depo-Provera® injection tends to stop bleeding over the long term. Using extended-cycle oral contraception or vaginal rings reduces blood loss as well.

Nearly all reproductive-aged women have experienced symptoms of premenstrual syndrome (PMS), which may include cramps, headaches, bloating, fatigue, acne, and other symptoms. Research shows that PMS and/or painful periods may lead girls and women to miss school or work, which may, in turn, be a factor in the gender wage gap. Painful periods or dysmenorrhea can produce menstrual contractions comparable to intrauterine pressure in the second stage of labor (Nelson & Shulman, 2018). According to Nelson and Shulman (2018), menstrual suppression is effective in treating PMS and painful periods. Hormonal contraception, including hormonal IUDs, the implant, the shot, the pill, and the ring, have been used off-label (i.e., in a manner meant to utilize its side effects) to successfully reduce menstrual cramping. In particular, extended cycles of oral contraception or vaginal rings can be particularly effective because they avoid bleeding altogether. Combined OCPs containing drospirenone, such as Yaz®, have been approved by the FDA to treat premenstrual dysphoric disorder (PMDD), which is more severe than PMS and causes depression and/or anxiety.

The FDA has approved Ortho Tri-Cyclen®, Estrostep®, and Yaz® specifically for treating moderate acne in menstruating women older than 14 years who need contraception. Research shows that other birth control options may be effective at treating acne as well. As a result, health-care providers may prescribe other hormonal contraceptive methods, including combined oral contraceptives and the vaginal ring, to help improve acne. Excess sebum, an oil, is one factor that causes acne. Hormonal contraception that contains estrogen and progesterone can lessen production of sebum and reduce acne. It may take a few months for an oral contraceptive to help clear acne, and health-care providers may prescribe additional forms of acne treatment in conjunction with birth control pills.

Does hormonal contraception treat or prevent pelvic inflammatory disease, polycystic ovarian syndrome, fibroids, and/or endometriosis?

PID is caused by sexually transmitted infections traveling into the uterus and fallopian tubes. We have discussed the defective Dalkon Shield, which was an IUD that caused PID before being taken off the market. Today, hormonal IUDs may actually protect against PID and uterine infections by thickening cervical mucus, which creates a barrier against infections. Women using oral contraception for at least 12 months have a lower risk of PID while they use the pill. Among women who do not want to become pregnant, hormonal contraception may be used to treat PCOS. Although there is no cure for PCOS, the hormonal IUD, OCP, the patch, the vaginal ring, the implant, and the shot may help to regulate periods, decrease excess hair growth, and improve acne.

Approximately one out of five women over 30 years of age has fibroids, which are benign uterine tumors. Most women do not notice they have fibroids. However, some women will have symptoms, such as pain, constipation, or abnormal bleeding. Among women trying to become pregnant, fibroids can cause miscarriage. Hormonal IUDs and the shot reduce bleeding and may shrink fibroids. The OCP or the ring may also be used to reduce bleeding.

There is no cure for endometriosis, which occurs when tissue similar to the uterine lining migrates to places other than the uterus; however, hormonal contraception can help to reduce pain and preserve fertility. In particular, birth control that ceases menstruation can reduce symptoms and halt the spread of the disease, which may increase the chance of a successful pregnancy. Extended cycles of hormonal IUDs, the OCP, the shot, or the vaginal ring may be used to treat endometriosis. The Depo-Provera® shot has been approved by the FDA for the treatment of pain related to endometriosis. According to Nelson and Shulman (2018), the contraceptive implant is as effective as the shot in treating pain related to endometriosis. Clinical trials have shown that hormonal IUDs are effective in treating pain and reducing the size of endometriotic lesions. A comparative trial showed that the vaginal ring reduced pain more successfully than oral contraceptives when both were used continuously without breaks. Research shows that progestin-only pills that suppress ovulation are more successful in treating endometriosis than combined OCPs (Nelson & Shulman, 2018).

Does hormonal contraception offer any health benefits?

In 2010, another study from the Royal College of General Practitioners' Oral Contraception Study investigated mortality risk among users of the OCP (Hannaford et al., 2010). Researchers found that women who had ever used oral contraception had a significantly lower rate of death from any cause. Findings were based on observing women for up to 39 years. Furthermore, women who had ever used oral contraception had significantly lower rates of death from all cancers, including gynecological cancers, such as ovarian and uterine body cancer, large bowel/rectum cancer, and all circulatory disease, including ischemic heart disease. In brief, researchers found a net health benefit among ever users of oral contraception, even in health areas that may traditionally concern women taking the birth control pill, such as cancer, heart disease, and stroke.

Another long-term cohort study, the Oxford–Family Planning Association contraceptive study, started in 1968. A 2010 analysis found that the use of oral contraception slightly reduced all-cause mortality among women (Vessey, Yeates, & Flynn, 2010). Researchers found that there was no association between mortality from breast cancer and ever-use of oral contraception. Using oral contraception did not increase circulatory disease mortality, either. Use of oral contraception strongly protected women against death from uterine and ovarian cancer. In fact, protection increased with longer oral contraception use and persisted longer than 20 years after stopping the birth control pill.

Does hormonal contraception prevent cancer?

Hormonal contraception has been shown to prevent colon, ovarian, and endometrial cancer. In 2017, researchers analyzed 44 years of follow up from the Royal College of General Practitioners' Oral Contraception Study (Iversen, Sivasubramaniam, Lee, Fielding, & Hannaford, 2017). The results related to breast cancer are described earlier in this chapter. The authors concluded that women who use oral contraception are likely to be protected from cancer in the long term. This analysis found that women who use oral contraception are protected from colorectal, endometrial, and ovarian cancer for up to 35 years or more after discontinuing the pill. Researchers again found that any increased breast and cervical cancer risk among current and recent users dissipated within about five years of discontinuing oral contraception. An unrelated random-effects meta-analysis published in *Obstetrics & Gynecology* found that women who had used an IUD experienced one-third less cervical cancer than those who did not use an IUD (Cortessis et al., 2017). Although these studies are not clinical trials, they provide a global pattern of evidence suggesting that hormonal contraception offers a net health benefit to women.

Is it safe to use birth control during perimenopause?

Healthy women who do not have hypertension, diabetes, cardiovascular risks, or other contraindications to estrogen may safely use combined oral contraception until menopause (Cwiak & Edelman, 2018). In addition to preventing unintended pregnancy, hormonal contraception during perimenopause provides cycle control, decreased blood loss, treatment of hot flashes and night sweats, some protection against bone loss, and reduction in the risk of certain cancers (Black & Nelson, 2018). Experts recommend that women in this age group receive regular health care to ensure that health issues that may develop with age are identified because certain conditions may increase the risk of using a contraceptive method with estrogen. According to Black and Nelson (2018), using OCPs and vaginal rings on an extended cycle will help women avoid bleeding, hot flashes, and night sweats. In addition, the vaginal ring increases lubrication and can relieve vaginal dryness and pain during sexual activity.

Is birth control recommended during the postpartum period?

Birth control is recommended during the postpartum period because research shows that birth to conception intervals (the time elapsed between birth of one child and conception of another) shorter than 18 months result in health complications for women and infants. Birth to conception intervals shorter than 12 months are associated with significant risks of preterm delivery and low birth weight. Research shows that women were 1.6 times more likely to avoid short birth to conception intervals if they received contraception in the post-partum period (Thiel de Bocanegra, Chang, Menz, Howell, & Darney, 2013).

There are a number of contraceptive options available to women in the postpartum period. In most cases, hormonal and nonhormonal IUDs can be inserted immediately following a vaginal or cesarean delivery. The implant and the birth control injection (or shot) can also be inserted right after delivery. Combined hormonal contraception methods that contain estrogen and progestin, such as birth control pills, the vaginal ring, and the patch should not be used in the first three weeks following delivery because of the increased risk of blood clots after childbirth. Women with additional risk factors for blood clots may be advised to wait up to six weeks after delivery to use combined hormonal methods. Finally, women can choose the mini-pill or progestin-only birth control pill, which contains only progestin.

Are hormonal contraceptives safe during breastfeeding?

Many women are concerned about the impact of hormonal contraceptive options on breastfeeding, including milk supply. According to one woman, "I probably wouldn't want to go on any contraception that is hormone-based while I'm breastfeeding." Other women described conflicting advice from healthcare providers about hormonal contraception and their ability to breastfeed. One woman described feeling persuaded not to choose the implant: "When I was actually in there having the baby, [the nurses] came in like five times and said, 'So are you sure you're getting the Nexplanon® in your arm when you get done?'" Many women have chosen the mini-pill or progestin-only birth control pill because it was believed that estrogen could negatively impact milk production. However, according to ACOG, studies of hormonal contraception have not shown a negative impact on breastfeeding, be it in terms of milk supply or breastfeeding duration.

Do I need to have a period?

People who menstruate do not need to have a period. The menstrual cycle typically lasts about 28 days. During the menstrual cycle, ovulation or the releasing of an egg occurs. If the egg is fertilized and implants in the lining of the uterus, a pregnancy results. Before ovulation occurs, the body releases hormones that increase the lining of the uterus in preparation for the implanting of a fertilized egg. If there is no pregnancy, the uterine lining is not needed and is shed during menstruation. When this blood and tissue exit the body, most people call it "a period."

Birth control regulates hormones, stopping ovulation, preventing the uterine lining from building up, and avoiding menstruation altogether. When people on hormonal birth control take one week of inactive or placebo pills or remove the vaginal ring for one week, for example, this causes withdrawal bleeding. Withdrawal bleeding is not a period. It results from a drop in the level of hormones in the body—not the passing of a menstrual cycle without pregnancy. Since hormonal contraception prevents the uterine lining from building up, it does not need to be shed if there is no pregnancy. In other words, without hormones that build up the uterine lining, there is no need to have a period.

Hormonal contraception allows people who menstruate to alter or avoid their menstrual cycle. The traditional OCP was originally designed with 21 days of active hormone pills and 7 days of placebo pills. When taking the placebo pills, women experience withdrawal bleeding, which mimics the symptoms of a period but, as we explained before, is not a period. Today, there are many more options that offer women the opportunity to shorten their withdrawal bleeding by taking 24 days of active hormone pills and 4 days of placebo pills, three months of active pills without any placebo pills, or extended cycle regimens that can stop bleeding for a year or longer. Many women stop having withdrawal bleeding when using IUDs, the implant, or the shot. This is perfectly healthy. There is no need for women to bleed regularly. As we previously described, continuous or extended cycles of oral contraceptives, the ring, or the patch, for example, offer many benefits related to heavy menstrual bleeding, PMS, cramps, headaches, anemia, etc. The only downside to avoiding withdrawal bleeding is the increased likelihood of unscheduled bleeding and spotting; however, this usually stops over time.

Some people who menstruate desire a "natural" cycle with moderation, including the ability to control timing and frequency of withdrawal bleeding. A recent study found that 38% of participants regularly altered their cycle and 73% had skipped pill-free intervals (Picavet, 2014). Another study found increasing numbers of college-aged women alter withdrawal bleeding for less frequent cycles (Lakehomer, Kaplan, Wozniak, & Minson, 2013). One woman we talked with described the nuance of this common perspective, "The pill is good for knowing when you are going to get your period, and you can skip a period. It's not bad, but it's not good. I've heard that it's not good for you. It's probably not good. But the doctor said it's not bad." Other women described the benefits of avoiding menstruation altogether, "I didn't have a problem not having a menstrual cycle. I liked not having one. I wasn't worried." Although there is no reason to have a period, social and cultural beliefs about reproductive health impact women's understanding of menstruation and the role of contraception in limiting or avoiding a monthly period.

Is there a medical reason to have a period every month?

There is no medical or health reason to have a period every month. When using hormonal contraception, studies show that there is no medical reason to have a monthly pill-free interval, which leads to withdrawal bleeding (Hillard, 2014; Picavet, 2014). A Cochrane Database Systematic Review, which is known as the gold standard of systematic reviews, reinforced the safety of extended cycle use of hormonal contraception, which offers increased satisfaction, fewer menstrual symptoms, fewer menstruation-related absences, and increased compliance (Edelman, Micks, Gallo, Jensen, & Grimes, 2014). Hormonal contraception prevents the lining of the uterus from thickening, so there is nothing to shed each month. Even though medical professionals agree that there is no reason to have a monthly period, some women have received contradictory advice from their health-care providers. According to one woman, "a nurse and a doctor told me that it is unhealthy to not have a menstrual cycle."

Why do many types of hormonal birth control attempt to mimic a "natural" 28-day cycle?

In the 1940s, chemist Russell Marker discovered Mexican wild yams, cabeza de negro, could be used to develop synthetic progesterone, which became the foundation for hormonal contraception. Gregory Pincus and John Rock at the Worcester Foundation for Experimental Biology, the creators of the OCP, conducted a fertility study with 50 women in the 1950s to test hormonal contraception. The FDA approved Enovid oral contraception in 1957 to treat severe menstrual disorders (not as a form of birth control), carrying the warning that it suppresses ovulation. Rock and Pincus created the 21-day hormonal cycle to mimic the "natural" process of menstruation. This decision was likely made in an effort to gain the approval of the Catholic Church, which did not happen (Gladwell, 2000). As a Catholic, John Rock was concerned that the OCP be accepted by the Pope. He believed that mirroring the natural 28-day menstrual cycle would be consistent with the church's teachings regarding natural family planning. It may also have been an effort to gain women's acceptance by mirroring their current lived experience.

This decision, made over 60 years ago, continues to reverberate in the social and cultural norms of hormonal contraceptive use. Many women describe using hormonal contraception to manage menstruation. According to one woman, "I've had doctors that have recommended me going on birth control pills before because my period is so erratic so I know that there are other benefits to them besides just the pregnancy prevention." Many women express a preference for contraceptive methods that mimic a natural menstrual cycle. One woman said, "I think it's not healthy, not normal [to skip a period]." Another woman said, "even though I learned you don't really need a period, I like to get it because it is maintaining a connection with my body." However, even women who prefer a natural cycle often describe moderating their cycle for special events: "You have a period once a month for a reason, but once or twice a year [skipping your period] won't kill you."

Although many women believe that it is "natural" and "healthy" to get a period, they may not be aware that the 21-day hormonal cycle was not based on scientific evidence. Indeed, from an evolutionary perspective, until the demographic transition, most women experienced many pregnancies and lactational amenorrhea resulting from extended breastfeeding. That means that women in a preindustrial society menstruated only 100 times in their life compared to an average of 350 to 400 times for the average American woman (Strassmann, 1999). Scholars suggest that this type of incessant menstruation is not "natural" and may be to blame for modern diseases, such as anemia, endometriosis, PMS, ovarian cancer, and endometrial cancer (Coutinho & Segal, 1999).

If I am using hormonal birth control, why do I have "withdrawal bleeding" for one week every month?

Most oral contraceptive options today are based on the traditional OCP developed by Rock and Pincus in the 1950s. Designed to mimic a "natural" menstrual cycle, the traditional birth control pill pack includes 21 hormonal pills and 7 inactive

or placebo pills. The week that you take the inactive or placebo pills causes withdrawal bleeding. Withdrawal bleeding
is a result of withdrawing or stopping the hormones—not the
passing of a menstrual cycle without pregnancy. Women can
avoid withdrawal bleeding by skipping the placebo pills and
starting a new pack of hormonal pills, or inserting a new vaginal ring. Withdrawal bleeding is not the same as a menstrual
period. Hormonal contraception prevents ovulation and keeps
the uterine lining thin, so the endometrium does not need to
be shed.

What is the difference between menstruation and "withdrawal bleeding?"

Menstruation and withdrawal bleeding are not the same.
Similar to menstruation, however, withdrawal bleeding results
from a drop in the level of hormones in the body. During a menstrual cycle, the drop in hormones would signal that there is no
pregnancy, causing the uterus to shed the blood and tissue that
had built up to support a fertilized egg. Withdrawal bleeding
is caused by a drop in hormones from not taking active birth
control. Since birth control prevents ovulation and stops the
uterine lining from building up, there is nothing that needs to
be shed. As a result, withdrawal bleeding is often lighter than
menstruation and may ultimately stop when using some contraception methods.

Does the presence of "withdrawal bleeding" mean I'm not pregnant?

No, the presence of withdrawal bleeding does not guarantee
that you are not pregnant. Many women we have talked with
resisted menstrual suppression based on the incorrect belief that withdrawal bleeding was the same as menstruation.
These women noted that "even when people are on the pill,
they are still worried about pregnancy." Monthly withdrawal
bleeding served as a "reassurance," and "getting your period

is good, it is reaffirming. If I didn't get it, I would get scared." One woman said:

> Different forms of the pill where you only get your period every 3 or 4 months, are not as popular. People who are sexually active want to get their period. They want a monthly, regular cycle, every time. They are reassured every month that the pill is fully effective.

These women found a "regular cycle" reassuring, even though withdrawal bleeding is unrelated to pregnancy—and withdrawal bleeding can still occur in cases of new pregnancy.

Withdrawal bleeding is caused by stopping the hormone progesterone. It is not a menstrual period because it is not the result of ovulation. Hormonal contraception maintains a steady level of hormones, which keeps the uterine lining thin. Since the uterine lining is thin, there is no build-up that needs to be shed. As a result, withdrawal bleeding is often lighter and shorter than a menstrual period. Since withdrawal bleeding is not a real menstrual period, it is also not a guarantee that you are not pregnant.

Is it healthy to alter my cycle if I am using hormonal birth control?

Yes, it is healthy to alter your cycle while using hormonal birth control. In 2019, the United Kingdom's Faculty of Sexual and Reproductive Healthcare (2019) issued contraceptive guidelines that strongly support skipping withdrawal bleeding, noting, "It should be made clear to women that this bleed does not represent physiological menstruation and that it is has no health benefit." Avoiding withdrawal bleeding may also be essential gender-affirming care of transgender individuals who experience gender dysphoria during bleeding.

According to Nelson and Shulman (2018), certain medical conditions, such as asthma, mental health disorders, and migraines, may worsen during a woman's menstrual cycle. For individuals who have medical conditions that are exacerbated by the menstrual cycle, menstrual suppression may be an essential noncontraceptive benefit of hormonal contraception (Allen & Cwiak, 2018). Menstrual suppression offered by contraception treats a number of medical conditions, including anemia, heavy menstrual bleeding, migraines, and painful periods. Furthermore, menstrual suppression may offer increased protection against ovarian and endometrial cancer (Allen & Cwiak, 2018).

4

BEYOND THE PILL

ARE THERE OTHER OPTIONS?

Almost 65% of U.S. women of reproductive age currently use a method of contraception, whether it's "the pill," patch, injection, vaginal ring, implant, intrauterine device (IUD), and/or condoms. Although research demonstrates that many women are dissatisfied with the pill, they remain uncertain about other birth control options. As a result, women's contraceptive needs continue to be unmet. Since 1982, female sterilization and the pill have been the most commonly used methods of birth control in the United States (Guttmacher Institute, 2018). Contraceptive use differs based on age, race/ethnicity, education, and other factors. Among African American women who are at risk of unintended pregnancy, 83% currently use a method of contraception, compared to 91% of Latina and White women, and 90% of Asian women (Guttmacher Institute, 2018). As women pursue more higher education, use of the pill increases and female sterilization declines. However, use of long-acting reversible contraceptive (LARC) methods, including IUDs and the implant, does not differ based on education.

Although the number of women aged 15 to 44 choosing a LARC method remains relatively low, use of IUDs and the implant has increased fivefold since the early 2000s. In 2002, approximately 1.5% of women used a LARC method. By 2013, 7.2% of women used a LARC method. According to the latest data from the 2015–2017 National Survey of Family Growth, 10.3% of women relied on a LARC method (Daniels & Abma, 2018). Despite this modest increase in use, women continue to favor female sterilization (18.6%) and the pill (12.6%). Women aged 20 to 29 were more likely to choose LARC methods (13.1%) compared to other age groups (Daniels & Abma, 2018).

Globally, women in other countries are more likely to use LARC methods, with 27% of Norwegian women and 23% of French women using an IUD. Europe did not experience the devastation of the Dalkon Shield IUD in the 1970s because it was rarely prescribed by doctors in those countries. Although not uniformly free to women in Europe, the high cost of LARC methods in the United States before the Affordable Care Act may have also been a powerful deterrent. LARC methods are cost-effective over time; however, they require a high upfront investment. Today, LARC methods are free in most cases because of the Affordable Care Act. Studies show that when contraceptive options are free and women are offered comprehensive counseling, they overwhelmingly choose LARC methods. When they do, they report high satisfaction and continuation over 12 months.

Why do many people believe that the pill and condoms are the only or best forms of contraception available today?

In the United States, there has been a considerable increase in male condom use since 1982 when only 52% of women reported ever using condoms. By 2010, 93% of women reported ever using the male condom (Guttmacher Institute, 2018). According to the Guttmacher Institute (2018), four out of five women who have had sexual intercourse have used the pill. More than 25% of contraceptive users choose the pill, making it the most popular form of reversible contraception. The pill is more likely to be used by adolescents and young adults, never-married or cohabiting women, and women without children (Guttmacher Institute, 2018). According to the National Survey of Family Growth (2015–2017), women with a bachelor's degree or higher were more likely to use the pill. Furthermore, use of the pill was more common among non-Hispanic White women (14.9%) compared to Hispanic (9.2%) and African American women (8.3%) (Daniels & Abma, 2018).

In our research, women described the pill as the norm, which led them to believe it was more effective and safer than other options. Indeed, many women understood birth control as synonymous with the pill. One woman said, "When you think of birth control, you think of the pill." Another woman said, "Birth control means the pill." We have talked with many women who expressed concerns about newer methods of contraception that may not be safe or "fully tested." According to one woman, "I know enough people who have used the pill, it's more common. I would want to be on something that they know enough about, that they know about the side effects." Many women believe that the pill is the most effective method of birth control. One woman said, "The pill is the most effective, other methods are less popular, so they must be less effective." Another woman said, "All hormonal methods work the same, when used properly, they are equally effective." Media also impacted women's perceptions of effectiveness. One woman told us, "I think all birth control is supposed to work the same. They don't advertise what works better than another method."

In the popular sitcom *Friends* in the episode "The One Where Rachel Tells . . . ," the character Ross is shocked to learn that condoms are not 100% effective exclaiming, "What? What? What?!! Well they should put that on the box!!!" He later explains that he is "indignant! As a consumer!" (Epps, 2001). According to the Centers for Disease Control and Prevention (CDC), condoms are only 82% effective even when used correctly. In other words, across a year of regular use, condoms have an 18% failure rate. Both oral contraception and condoms are "user dependent," meaning they have relatively high failure rates with typical use—different than their hypothetical effectiveness in a controlled experimental setting. Typical use of the pill has a failure rate of 9%, meaning that it is only 91% effective. Furthermore, condoms and oral contraceptives have relatively low continuation rates—the degree to which users stick with them over time—which may be related to method dissatisfaction. A recent study found that continuation rates for oral contraception may be as low as 29% after six months (Gilliam et al., 2010). Research shows that LARC methods are more effective than the oral contraceptive pill (OCP) and condoms, as well as acceptable and easy to use for most women, including young adults.

Why do women feel that the pill is something that they can control?

Many women appreciate being "in control" of taking the pill everyday (Sundstrom, 2012). In interviews, some women have expressed satisfaction with being "responsible enough" to take the OCP at exactly the same time every day. One woman said, "You must be very organized and responsible to take it every day." Women, especially young women, developed community-based cultural norms around taking the pill, including setting a cell phone alarm as a reminder to take it at the same time every day. Some groups of friends provided additional social support to remind each other to take the pill by setting a phone alarm at the same time as their friends. Women who chose nondaily contraceptive options were perceived as irresponsible. One woman said, "I don't think other people are as serious as I am about taking it at the same time every day." In this way, taking the pill every day is something that women can control and reinforces their identity as "organized," "responsible," and "serious."

Many women believe that the pill offers them control over their menstrual cycle. As we discussed in Chapter 3 of this book, the pill's traditional 28-day cycle includes a week of placebo pills that allows withdrawal bleeding to occur. This is not a menstrual period because birth control prevents ovulation and stops the uterine lining from building up, so there is nothing that needs to be shed. However, many women believe withdrawal bleeding is the same as a menstrual period. In our research, as we discussed in Chapter 3, women expressed their desire for a natural cycle with some modification. Many women believe that the pill provides the ability to control frequency and timing of monthly periods.

What is the myth of perfect use?

With "perfect use," such as in a laboratory or clinical setting, the OCP is 99% effective. Typical use reflects the rate of unintended pregnancies among all individuals taking the pill. With typical use, the OCP is only 91% effective. This accounts for how women take the pill in everyday life, which may include missing pills, forgetting to take it at the same time every day, and possible interactions with certain supplements and medications (prescribed and over the counter) that may make the pill less effective.

In our research, many women described struggling to take the pill at the same time every day, including forgetting to take a pill at the right time or missing a pill. One woman said, "If I forget, I freak out that it doesn't work the same." According to one young woman, "a lot of people forget, especially in college, your lifestyle doesn't make it easy to take [it] at the same time every day." Many women even knew of someone who became pregnant while taking the pill. Still, in our research, women expected "perfect use" effectiveness for themselves. They believed that the pill could be 99% effective in everyday life. In other words, they described a myth of perfect use whereby they wanted to be in control by taking the pill every day despite imperfect adherence (Sundstrom, Baker-Whitcomb, & DeMaria, 2015). The myth of perfect use impacted how they perceived the effectiveness of the OCP. In fact, some women suggested that perfect daily adherence offered increased control over the method's effectiveness. This led some women to view LARC methods with skepticism because they were not in control of taking it every day.

What is the paradox of inertia?

The paradox of inertia is the tendency to remain on the pill despite strong external forces, such as dissatisfaction, forgetting to take the pill on time, and recognizing LARC as a better option. In talking with women about their birth control practices, a pattern emerged: as the pill becomes part of women's identities and reinforces positive qualities such as responsibility, women are less likely to choose other contraceptive options. The myth of perfect use and women's desire for control when choosing a contraceptive method led to what we coined the paradox of inertia (Sundstrom, Billings & Zenger, 2016). Many women described dissatisfaction with the pill, including forgetting to take it on time. Most women were familiar with LARC methods and could describe the benefits of these options, even suggesting that LARC was a better choice. Despite this knowledge, women resisted switching to a LARC method, creating a paradox of inertia. The paradox of inertia helps us to understand the strength of the pill as a social norm, the importance of control and responsibility in contraceptive choice, and the myths and misconceptions surrounding LARC methods. The paradox of inertia explains why women haven't simply switched to a LARC method based on the recommendations of experts.

What birth control methods do the experts recommend?

The American College of Obstetricians and Gynecologists (ACOG) recommends LARC methods as the best, first-line contraceptive options for all women and adolescents. ACOG first established this best practice in 2012 and strengthened their recommendation in 2015. The American Academy of

Pediatrics (AAP) concurred with this recommendation in 2014, establishing IUDs and the implant as the best options for adolescents and young women. ACOG and AAP agree that LARC methods are safe and effective for all women without limitation based on age or whether they have given birth. LARC methods, including IUDs and the implant are user-independent and more than 99% effective. They can last a long time; however, women may remove them at any time. According to ACOG, LARC methods offer one solution to the problem of unintended pregnancy.

What are long-acting reversible contraceptive methods?

LARC methods include IUDs and the implant. In the United States, women have access to five IUDs and one arm implant. IUDs include hormonal and nonhormonal options. There are four hormonal IUDs, including Mirena®, Skyla®, Liletta®, and Kyleena®, which last between three and five years. ParaGard® is the only nonhormonal IUD available in the United States and can last for up to 10 years. The Nexplanon® arm implant is a small rod that's inserted in the skin of the upper arm and releases progestin to prevent pregnancy for up to three years.

How do LARC methods work?

The IUD is a tiny piece of plastic shaped like a T. IUDs are inserted in the uterus by a trained clinician, eliminating the possibility of user error. IUDs are well-liked by women with high rates of continuation and satisfaction. Once inserted, women (and their partners) should not be able feel the IUD. Short strings from the IUD hang into the vagina so that women can check to make sure the IUD remains in place. In our research, one woman said, "I love that it's a very discrete and powerful birth control without having to take a daily pill." IUDs offer hormonal and nonhormonal options. The ParaGard® IUD does not contain hormones. It is made of plastic and natural, safe copper. It works by stopping sperm from reaching and fertilizing the egg. It is approved for use up to 10 years; however, recent studies show that it is effective for up to 12 years.

Hormonal IUDs available in the United States include Mirena®, Skyla®, Liletta®, and Kyleena®. These IUDs are made of plastic and prevent pregnancy by releasing the hormone progestin (they do not contain estrogen). Since IUDs are placed in the uterus, smaller amounts of progestin circulate through the blood stream compared to the pill. Hormonal IUDs work by thickening cervical mucus to prevent sperm from reaching the uterus, impacting sperm's ability to move, and stopping ovulation. Hormonal IUDs are approved for use from three to five years; however, recent studies show that they can last between three and six years, depending on the type.

The implant is the most effective method of reversible contraception available today. In our research, one woman said about the implant, "It's stress-free birth control. You don't have to think about it." The implant is a single, thin rod that is inserted by a trained clinician under the skin of the upper arm. It takes about one minute to insert it and about three minutes to remove it. The implant releases the hormone progestin, which prevents pregnancy by stopping ovulation and thickening cervical mucus to prevent sperm from reaching the uterus. Although Nexplanon® has been approved for use up to three years, recent studies show that it is effective for up to four years.

Why are LARC methods considered the first-line contraceptive recommendation for all women?

In 2015, ACOG strengthened its recommendation of LARC methods as the first-line contraceptive option for all women and adolescents in part because they are the most effective forms of reversible contraception. LARC methods are safe for most women and can be removed at any time. Moreover, women can get pregnant immediately after removal of these methods. Since LARC methods are inserted by a trained clinician, they do not require regular user adherence and eliminate the possibility of user error. As a result, the effectiveness of these methods is not linked to sexual activity, user motivation, or adherence. In addition to effectiveness, LARC methods also offer the highest continuation and user satisfaction rates compared to other options, which is essential for contraceptive success.

Studies from one cohort study, the Contraceptive CHOICE Project, found that improving knowledge of and access to LARC methods increased use and decreased unintended pregnancies and abortions, including among adolescents (McNicholas, Tessa, Secura, & Peipert, 2014). LARC methods eliminate the need for frequent visits to the pharmacy and to the doctor's office for yearly prescription renewals. As a result, LARC methods are cost-effective over the long term. For most women, LARC methods should be free because of the Affordable Care Act. Studies show that health-care providers are much more likely to choose LARC methods for themselves compared to the 10.3% of U.S. women who rely on a LARC (Daniels & Abma, 2018). One recent study found that 42% of female health-care providers in a national sample used a LARC method (Stern et al., 2015). The authors suggested that knowledge and access likely played a role in this difference.

Are LARC methods effective?

LARC methods are the most effective methods of reversible contraception available. They are more than 99% effective in preventing pregnancy. That means that there will be less than one unintended pregnancy out of every 100 women using the method within the first year of typical use. The implant is the most effective method of reversible contraception with a failure rate of 0.05%, making it 99.95% effective. Hormonal IUDs have a failure rate of 0.2%, making them 99.8% effective. The nonhormonal IUD has a failure rate of 0.8%, making it 99.2% effective. Among participants in the Contraceptive CHOICE Project, LARC methods were 20 times more effective at preventing pregnancy than the OCP, patch, or ring.

Are LARC methods easy to access and use?

In general, LARC methods require an office visit and trained clinician to insert and remove. However, despite headlines such as "No, You Should Absolutely Not Remove Your IUD at Home," research shows that it is possible for women to remove their own IUDs. While it is preferable to visit a trained clinician for IUD removal, this may be a barrier to use for some women. The IUD Removal Options Study found that counseling women on the option of IUD self-removal may increase interest in the method and empower women facing barriers to removal (Raifman, Barar, & Foster, 2018).

In 2015, ACOG provided guidance to clinicians to increase access to LARC methods. Best practices include offering IUDs and the implant the same day as requested, as well as at the time of delivery, abortion, or treatment for miscarriage. ACOG recommends treating sexually transmitted infections (STIs) without removal of the IUD and offering the copper IUD as the most effective method of emergency contraception. Another potential barrier to accessing LARC methods is cost. In general, LARC methods have relatively high up-front costs but are cost-effective over time. In the United States, LARC methods should be free because of the Affordable Care Act. Most health insurance plans are required by law to cover all U.S. Food and Drug Administration (FDA)-approved methods of birth control, including IUDs and the implant. However, there are exceptions, and some plans don't cover all brands of IUDs. There are a number of state-run programs and pharmaceutical patient assistance programs that may provide LARC methods at low or no cost to eligible individuals. Health-care providers can direct patients to appropriate resources in their state.

How does the history of the Dalkon Shield impact opinions about the IUD today?

In the 1970s, the Dalkon Shield was a malfunctioning IUD that increased the risk of pelvic inflammatory disease (PID) and infertility. Following devasting health impacts on women, the manufacturer voluntarily discontinued sale of the Dalkon Shield IUD in 1974. The Dalkon Shield controversy led to an immediate and long-term decline in all IUD use among U.S. women until at least 1988. Rates remained stable and very low until recently. According to the National Survey of Family Growth, in 2002, among women aged 15 to 44 who had ever had sexual intercourse, 5.8% reported ever using an IUD. Between 2011 and 2015, 15% of women reported ever using an IUD. Despite recent increases, use of IUDs remains very low considering it is the first-line contraception option for all women.

What are the side effects of LARC methods?

There are many positive side effects of LARC methods. IUDs are easy to use, independent of sexual intercourse, private, long-lasting, compatible with breastfeeding, and may be a safer option for smokers and those with certain health conditions. Hormonal IUDs may reduce cramps and menstrual bleeding. Some women may have negative side effects when using an IUD, including cramps, backaches, and spotting between periods. Users of the copper IUD often experience increased menstrual bleeding, which usually decreases over time. Serious side effects are rare but may include the IUD falling out, infection, or the IUD attaching to or piercing the wall of the uterus.

The implant is easy to use, independent of sexual intercourse, private, long-lasting, and compatible with breastfeeding. It may be a safer option for women who can't take estrogen, smokers, and those with certain health conditions.

Women using the implant typically have fewer, lighter periods. Some women may have negative side effects when using an implant. The most common side effect is irregular bleeding, which may include spotting, longer, heavier bleeds, or no bleeding at all. Some women have reported a change in appetite, headache, acne, and depressed mood.

Does the insertion of LARC methods hurt?

Pain is subjective and often varies between individuals. It is important to know that women can talk with their health-care providers about managing pain before insertion of a LARC method. In most cases, insertion of the implant is quick and easy. A trained clinician numbs a small area of the upper arm and inserts the implant under the skin. It takes about one minute to insert it. We have heard, "You've cut yourself shaving worse than this!" To remove it, a provider numbs the arm, makes a tiny incision in the skin and takes the implant out. A new implant can be inserted at the same time. Removal takes about three minutes.

Pain during IUD insertion varies widely. For many women, especially those who have given birth, IUD insertion may feel like getting a Pap test. For some women, IUD insertion may cause very strong cramps. In our research, one woman described IUD insertion as "the worst period cramps ever." Insertion usually lasts less than five minutes. One woman we talked with described the trade-off as "short-term pain, long-term gain." The news media may sensationalize the likelihood of experiencing significant pain during IUD insertion. Recent headlines include "Why IUD Insertions Are So Incredibly Painful" from the *Huffington Post* (Birch, 2019) and "Pain on a Cosmic Level: Getting an IUD Can Be Excruciating. Is There a Better Way?" from *Slate* (Cauterucci, 2015).

Health-care providers may recommend taking an over-the-counter pain killer, such as ibuprofen, before an IUD insertion. Scheduling an IUD insertion during menstruation can help because the cervix is already slightly open. Health-care providers may also offer a local numbing medicine that is injected into the cervix. In the past, health-care providers prescribed a medicine to soften the cervix prior to IUD insertion; however, recent research concluded that these drugs did not help with pain. Many women are able to return to their normal activities immediately after insertion, while others may experience cramping for a few days. A follow-up appointment will be scheduled to make sure the IUD stays in the right place.

How do LARC methods impact menstruation?

The copper IUD does not contain hormones, so it does not interfere with the menstrual cycle. However, women may experience worse cramping and heavier bleeding for six months following insertion. Then, the menstrual cycle should return to normal. Women using hormonal IUDs may experience irregular bleeding for approximately six months followed by lighter bleeding or no bleeding at all. Approximately one in five people stop bleeding entirely after one year. According to the Contraceptive CHOICE Project, women who already have lighter or moderate periods are more likely to stop bleeding completely. The implant may cause irregular bleeding at first followed by reduced cramping and lighter bleeding or no bleeding at all. Approximately one in three people stop bleeding at all after one year. As we discussed in Chapter 3 of this book, it is completely safe to stop getting a period while using hormonal contraception. Hormonal contraception prevents ovulation and keeps the uterine lining thin, so the endometrium does not need to be shed.

How do LARC methods protect fertility?

After LARC methods are removed, women return to being able to become pregnant immediately. Most women ovulate two weeks after stopping hormonal contraception, which means they can become pregnant before having a period. Studies show that one-year pregnancy rates among women stopping LARC methods are comparable to women using other contraceptive options or no contraception at all. As we discussed in Chapter 3 of this book, some LARC methods may also protect fertility by limiting unnecessary ovulations. Limiting ovulation is also the mechanism by which hormonal contraception decreases the risk of ovarian cancer.

Are LARC methods safe for women?

ACOG and AAP agree that LARC methods are safe for almost all women without limitation based on age or whether they have given birth. In fact, LARC methods may be a safer option for smokers and those with certain health conditions. Furthermore, recent research shows that women who had used an IUD experienced one third less cervical cancer than those who did not use an IUD (Cortessis et al., 2017).

Are LARC methods safe for adolescents?

IUDs and implants are safe for adolescents. Complications of LARC methods are rare and are not more likely among adolescents compared with older women. ACOG, the American Academy of Pediatrics, the Society of Family Planning, and the CDC recommend LARC methods for adolescents. In many, although not all, states, adolescents have the right to receive contraception, including IUDs and the implant, without parental consent. Hormonal contraception offers adolescents the same health benefits as women, including treating or preventing anemia, heavy menstrual bleeding and cramps, acne, migraines, PID, ovarian cysts, polycystic ovarian syndrome, uterine fibroids (myomata), endometriosis, uterine cancer, endometrial cancer, ovarian cancer, and colon cancer.

For more information on the health benefits of contraception, see Chapter 3 of this volume.

Adolescents report high satisfaction and continuation rates with LARC methods (Rosenstock, Peipert, Madden, Zhao, & Secura, 2012). The Contraceptive CHOICE Project found that adolescents were more likely to still be using LARC methods after one year compared to short-acting contraception, such as the pill (Secura et al., 2010). This same study found that adolescents using LARC methods were significantly less likely to have an unintended pregnancy (Secura et al., 2014). As we have seen with adults, adolescents who received comprehensive contraceptive counseling and could choose any method of contraception at no cost were more likely to choose a LARC method (Mestad et al., 2011). Still, according to the latest data from the 2015–2017 National Survey of Family Growth, only 8.2% of women aged 15 to 19 relied on a LARC method (Daniels & Abma, 2018).

According to ACOG's (2018a) latest committee opinion, IUDs are safe for adolescents and have very low rates of complications, including PID and uterine perforation. The risk of PID is highest in the first 20 days after insertion; however, over time hormonal IUDs lower future risk of PID by thinning the endometrium and thickening cervical mucus (ACOG, 2018a). Research shows that expulsion of an IUD is not more likely among adolescents compared to other women. ACOG recommends that clinicians counsel adolescent patients that insertion of the Skyla® and Kyleena® IUD may be easier and less painful than the Mirena® IUD since they are smaller.

ACOG's (2018a) analysis of the current research finds that the contraceptive implant has minimal or no effect on adolescents' bone density or weight. Hormonal contraception will not impact growth after menstruation begins. Since adolescents are at a higher risk of STIs, ACOG (2018a) recommends that adolescents using LARC methods should also use male or female condoms to decrease the risk of STIs. However, research shows that adolescents are not more likely to start having sex after beginning contraception. In fact, studies show that contraceptive use may lead to teens making healthier, less risky choices about sexual behavior. Adolescents face some of the same barriers to LARC methods as other women, including lack of knowledge about these methods, high upfront cost, and lack of access. Teens may also face misconceptions about LARC use among adolescents by their parents or health-care providers (ACOG, 2018a).

Are LARC methods safe for women who have just had a baby?

LARC methods are safe and effective for women who have just had a baby. ACOG and the CDC recommend that the immediate postpartum period, when women are still in the hospital after delivering an infant, is a safe and effective time to provide contraception. In most cases, hormonal and nonhormonal IUDs can be inserted immediately following a vaginal or cesarean delivery. The implant and the birth control injection (or shot) can also be inserted right after delivery. According to ACOG, studies of hormonal contraception have not shown a negative impact on breastfeeding outcomes, such as milk supply or breastfeeding duration.

ACOG aims to ensure that women have access to all appropriate methods of contraception before leaving the hospital after childbirth. The ACOG LARC Program's Postpartum Contraceptive Access Initiative offers training for the delivery of immediate postpartum LARC methods. The Office of Population Affairs (OPA) at the U.S. Department of Health and Human Services developed a contraceptive care measure that includes postpartum access to LARC methods. While women should have access to LARC methods after childbirth, the OPA warns that given the historical coercive practices related to contraception, providers should not encourage high rates of use that may lead to coercion.

What do women think about LARC methods?

Research shows that when contraceptive options are free and women are offered comprehensive counseling, they overwhelmingly choose LARC methods and report high satisfaction and continuation over 12 months. In our research, women using LARC methods report being highly satisfied with IUDs and the implant. Many of these women described ease of use as their favorite aspect of LARC methods. One woman said she loved her LARC because, "I don't have to remember to take a pill at the same time every day." Another woman said, "I don't even have to think about it."

In our research, women received messages about LARC methods from the media and from their in person and online social networks (Sundstrom, 2015). Many women don't know someone who has personally used a LARC method. This is a challenge because women often rely on personal experiences and find the stories of women particularly helpful in making contraceptive decisions. According to one woman, "I want to hear from someone I trust and personally know, who has used the method." Most women receive contraceptive advice from their mothers, who may have misconceptions about the safety of IUDs because of the malfunctioning Dalkon Shield. According to one woman, "I talked to my mom, I definitely had a conversation with her, and she said the IUD was terrifying and unnecessary." The media also impacts women's understanding of LARC methods indirectly. For example, women accurately perceived that commercials about the Mirena® IUD catered to an "older generation" and women who already had children.

Why do some health-care providers not recommend LARC methods to their patients?

According to ACOG, about half of obstetrician-gynecologists offer the implant. Providers who do not offer the implant cite lack of patient interest and lack of clinician training for not providing the method. Although obstetrician-gynecologists typically provide IUDs in their practices, they may use unnecessarily strict criteria to determine if women are eligible for this method. Providers may not be familiar with all FDA-approved LARC methods and recent changes in practice guidelines. ACOG (2015) recommends that clinicians encourage consideration of LARC methods for all women, including adolescents and women who have not had a baby. Best practices for LARC insertion include providing IUDs and the implant the same day as requested and offering these methods immediately after childbirth, abortion, or treatment for miscarriage.

What options do health-care providers offer women who are seeking birth control?

In our research, many women described health-care providers prescribing the pill without providing comprehensive contraceptive counseling. One woman said, "My doctor didn't sit me down and discuss my options." Another woman told us that her doctor said, "I'm going to go ahead and write a prescription for the pill." In some cases, women specifically asked for the pill. According to one woman, "I went to the doctor saying I want the pill. The doctor recommended a pill and said, 'I'm going to prescribe you this'; she didn't mention other options" (Sundstrom, 2012).

Other women met resistance when asking about LARC methods. One woman said, "I got the idea [of the arm implant] from my sister, who is a nurse. . . . My doctor just said, 'It would probably be better for you to go on the pill.' I was like okay, fine." Some women were told they were too young for IUDs or the implant. Other women faced barriers to obtaining a LARC method, including requirements to make multiple appointments or initiate a different hormonal contraceptive option before insertion. According to one woman,

I wanted to change from the pill and asked [my doctor] for the IUD and she literally gave me a stack of information on everything I could possibly change to and then set up another appointment in a month and was like, "we will talk about it in a month." Great.

Lack of physician knowledge and barriers to insertion led some women to question if it would be difficult or costly to remove a LARC method (Sundstrom et al., 2016).

Why do some health-care providers resist providing some methods to young women or women who have not yet had a baby?

Health-care providers may have misconceptions about the safety of LARC methods for young women or women who have not yet had a baby. Other providers may not be trained to insert these methods. A recent study showed that almost one third of health-care providers had misconceptions about the safety of IUDs for women who had not yet had a baby (Tyler et al., 2012). In that same study, more than 60% of health-care providers rarely provided IUDs to women who had not yet had a baby. These misconceptions likely result from the history of IUDs in the United States and sociocultural expectations about young women's reproductive health. This hesitancy on the part of providers may make it more difficult for women to make the best contraceptive choices for themselves. Indeed, ACOG recommends that health-care providers counsel all women and adolescents to consider LARC methods as the best, first-line contraceptive option.

Do I need an annual exam to get a prescription for birth control?

In our research, many women described the challenges of an annual physician's appointment to obtain a prescription for birth control, including cost, transportation, child care, work conflicts, inconvenience, and embarrassment. These barriers led women to experience gaps in contraceptive use, which put them at risk of unintended pregnancy. According to the World Health Organization and ACOG, hormonal contraception can be prescribed without an annual exam. Although ACOG recommends an annual exam, it should not be used as a barrier to prescribing hormonal contraception. Furthermore, screening for cervical cancer (i.e., a Pap test) or STIs is not medically necessary to provide hormonal contraception (ACOG, 2012). In addition, a pelvic examination is not necessary before prescribing or starting contraception, except for an IUD (ACOG, 2018b).

In fact, experts are divided about whether healthy, low-risk, nonpregnant women ever need a pelvic exam at all. In 2014, a systematic review found that pelvic exams do not offer a health benefit and often cause discomfort, distress, and sometimes lead to unnecessary surgery. Based on this analysis, the American College of Physicians recommended that healthy, low-risk women did not need annual pelvic exams (Qaseem, Humphrey, Harris, Starkey, & Denberg, 2014). ACOG (2018b) recommends that pelvic exams be performed when women have symptoms or a medical history that warrants such examination. Without those conditions, the decision to perform a pelvic exam should be shared between the patient and provider (ACOG, 2018b).

Can a pharmacist prescribe hormonal contraception?

According to the National Alliance of State Pharmacy Associations, 93% of Americans live within five miles of a pharmacy. That makes pharmacies accessible to most women in the United States. For the first time in 2016, state laws in California and Oregon authorized pharmacists to prescribe hormonal contraception. Since then, Colorado, the District of Columbia, Hawaii, Idaho, Maryland, New Hampshire, New Mexico,

Tennessee, Utah, Washington, and West Virginia passed statutes or regulations allowing pharmacists to prescribe birth control. Once the laws go into effect, however, not all pharmacies in those states will automatically offer the service.

Some states may limit pharmacists to prescribing self-administered contraception (e.g., the pill, patch, and ring). Other places, such as Oregon, may allow pharmacists to prescribe and dispense user-dependent hormonal contraception, as well as the shot. Currently, pharmacies do not provide LARC methods. It is important to know that there may be age restrictions for women under age 18. Pharmacies may charge a visit fee, usually up to $50, for the consultation and prescription. Health insurance should still cover all FDA-approved methods of contraception with no copay. Since these laws are relatively new, individuals are encouraged to check with their local pharmacy directly to make sure the service is available. You can also find more information at https://www.birthcontrolpharmacies.com/.

Can I get a year supply of birth control?

In our research, women described struggling to refill their birth control prescriptions on time every month. Barriers to consistent contraceptive use included transportation challenges, changing work or school schedules and moving or leaving the area periodically. These struggles were exacerbated for women who live in rural areas. According to ACOG, contraceptive continuation rates are higher among women who are provided with multiple months of birth control at one time. Research shows that providing a year supply of birth control decreases unintended pregnancies by 30% and decreases abortion by 46% (Foster et al., 2011). Unfortunately, many health insurance plans limit birth control to a one-month or three-month supply.

The CDC and the OPA recommend providing a year of birth control to reduce gaps in contraceptive continuation.

Some states have passed laws that require health insurance companies to provide a year supply of birth control. The states that require insurance coverage of a year supply of birth control are California, Colorado, Hawaii, Illinois, Maine, Nevada, New York, Oregon, Vermont, Virginia, Washington, and Washington, DC. As a result of the Affordable Care Act, all FDA-approved contraceptive methods should be provided free without cost-sharing.

Are there studies that show women prefer LARC methods when cost is not an issue?

The Contraceptive CHOICE Project, one of the largest prospective cohort studies of contraceptive choice in the United States, found that when knowledge, access, and cost are not an issue, individuals are more likely to choose LARC methods (McNicholas et al., 2014). Women who chose LARC methods were also more likely to continue using them and be highly satisfied with their choice. Increasing uptake of LARC methods also led to decreases in unintended pregnancy and abortion (McNicholas et al., 2014).

Are there any communication campaigns that provide information or resources about LARC methods?

Communication campaigns serve a critical role in achieving the 2020 national objective to increase intended pregnancies to 56%. In particular, communication campaigns are well-positioned to address misconceptions about LARC methods, which offer an important opportunity to increase intended pregnancies. In recent years, national and local health communication campaigns have focused on improving women's method satisfaction to reduce unintended pregnancies. In 2011, the Ad Council, in partnership with the Power to Decide (formerly the National Campaign to Prevent Teen and Unplanned Pregnancy), designed the first national multimedia campaign to assist young people with identifying a method that best suits their life. Bedsider (bedsider.org) continues to offer an interactive online and mobile Birth Control Support Network providing in-depth content about all methods and recommending IUDs and the implant.

5

HOW DO ATTITUDES AND POLICIES IMPACT ACCESS TO BIRTH CONTROL?

What attitudes and beliefs affect access to birth control in the United States?

The vast majority of the American public believes birth control is a fundamental right that all people should have access to. This consensus has persisted for years: in 1937, 61% of Americans polled supported the birth control movement; decades later, in 2010, Americans responding to a poll about the birth control pill affirmed that most saw it as a benefit to families and societies. Half of those polled, in fact, said that the pill changed family life for the better. In a 2015 survey, when asked "if birth control in general was morally acceptable, 89% of the country said it was" (Weldon, 2014).

Despite this public support, women's health care policies, especially those related to contraception, remain controversial, with some religious groups, states, politicians, and organizations in the United States opposed to increasing access to affordable birth control or actively trying to decrease access to it. These individuals and groups affect public opinion as well as policy decisions and laws (Barrett, Da Vanzo, Ellison, & Grammich, 2014, p. 162).

It is important to note that attitudes concerning birth control change and transform given particular historical and cultural contexts. In fact, the existence of *any* widespread opposition to birth control in the United States is a relatively new historical and cultural phenomenon. In the 1950s and 1960s, not only the American public, but also the vast majority of elected officials from both political parties, supported the growing family planning movement and its advocacy of birth control (Aiken & Scott, 2016). Until the 1970s, most Americans, including religious and evangelical Protestants, favored contraception. But birth control became more contested in the 1980s, 1990s, and 2000s. This development coincided with broader religious and cultural movements promoting a new social conservatism marked by evangelical Protestantism, the rise of the "New Right," and a corresponding glorifying of the nuclear family and Christian motherhood (Barrett et al., 2014, p. 163).

Since the late twentieth century, a powerful antiabortion campaign, which sometimes incorrectly conflates abortion and birth control, also has affected popular views of family planning. A fervent antiabortion movement emerged in the wake of *Roe vs. Wade* (1973), the landmark Supreme Court ruling that decriminalized abortion nationwide. In response, a corresponding "prochoice" movement was formed, and in the decades since, opinions about abortion have become more and more polarized. The politicization of abortion in the United States from the 1970s to the present day has impacted policies about all aspects of women's health, including family planning.

Discussions about both contraception and abortion frequently are framed within larger debates about what is best for women, families, and society. These debates, in turn, often center on interpretations of the role of religion in American life. Anticontraception campaigns, for example, gained steam with the support of the Catholic Church in the mid- to late twentieth century. Responding to the creation of the birth control pill and perceptions that a more permissive sexual culture was rising in Europe and the United States, in 1968 Pope Paul VI published *Humanae Vitae*, a document that resolutely affirmed the Church's opposition to birth control. It reads, in part:

> Therefore We base Our words on the first principles of a human and Christian doctrine of marriage when We are obliged once more to declare that the direct interruption of the generative process already begun and, above all, all direct abortion, even for therapeutic reasons, are to be absolutely excluded as lawful means of regulating the number of children. Equally to be condemned, as the magisterium of the Church has affirmed on many occasions, is direct sterilization, whether of the man or of the woman, whether permanent or temporary. Similarly excluded is any action which either before, at the moment of, or after sexual intercourse, is specifically intended to prevent procreation—whether as an end or as a means. (Paul VI, 1968)

While the principles outlined in *Humanae Vitae* and the Catholic Church's steadfast opposition to "artificial" birth control remain unchanged, a majority of American Catholics use birth control. According to the Guttmacher Institute (2018), 89% of Catholics at risk of unintended pregnancy currently use a method of contraception. In fact, 68% of Catholics use a highly effective method (i.e., sterilization, hormonal contraception, or intrauterine device [IUD]), and only 2% rely on natural family planning. Official views and actual practices, then, do not always align.

In the 1970s and 1980s, certain American Protestant denominations also increased their opposition to birth control. Some evangelical Christian organizations combined forces with a New Right political conservatism, forming a powerful new political movement. This movement asserted that the United States is a Christian nation and, as such, must implement Christian values. According to some within the New Right,

Christianity has been under siege in American politics for decades. This "war on religion," claim some evangelicals, requires a concerted political response. Since the 1980s, sexuality and reproduction have featured prominently in this response. An extensive proabstinence campaign in the early 1990s, directed primarily at adolescents, denounced contraception, framing it as promoting promiscuity and linking it with abortion and moral decadence. Abstinence (or "purity") educational campaigns, often supported by federal funding, have urged teenagers to abstain from sex until marriage. These campaigns argue that by encouraging contraception use, American society has promoted sex before marriage. Citing the biblical dictate "be fruitful and multiply," some of these same evangelicals also oppose the use of all forms of birth control after marriage. According to Nancy Campbell, leader of the conservative Christian movement Quiverfull, "The womb is such a powerful weapon; it's a weapon against the enemy. . . . My greatest impact is through my children. The more children I have, the more ability I have to impact the world for God" (Hagerty, 2009). Citing Psalm 127:5, which claims that men whose quivers are full of children are blessed, Quiverfull Christians advocate unrestricted reproduction (after marriage) to populate the country with other evangelicals and thus combat what they perceive as an increasingly secular United States that is hostile to religious and moral values.

By interpreting attitudes toward birth control as a "war" on religion and using militaristic language, anticontraception activists and thinkers employ some of the same strategies of those who advocate *for* birth control. Feminist activists and women's health organizations argue that attacks on birth control amount to a "war on women." This war, they claim, has a long history in the United States. According to historian Rickie Solinger (2013), "debates about who should have the power to manage women's reproductive capacities have often been linked to debates involving larger issues—social, cultural, and economic, across the spectrum" (p. 18). Within this context,

Solinger reminds us, women have often been "excluded from . . . rule-making processes" (p. 18). In the twentieth century and today, feminist activists have argued that "women's health, safety, dignity, and access to full citizenship depend[s] on their ability to control their own bodies and fertility" (p. 19). Opponents of the "war on women" link bodily autonomy with rights and citizenship, demanding policies and laws that protect practices such as contraception and abortion.

During the 2012 U.S. election and thereafter, when some Republican legislators came out in opposition to the Affordable Care Act's (ACA) contraceptive mandate (discussed later in this chapter), some Democratic politicians bemoaned that there was still a "war on women" being perpetuated by Republicans. After Barack Obama won the White House for a second term in 2012, polls and studies affirmed that women voters, possibly responding to a perceived attack on contraception and larger "war on women," were largely responsible for this victory (Deckman & McTague, 2015).

As we discussed in Chapter 2 of this book, popular attitudes toward birth control in the United States are also informed by history and culture. The history of "coercion, cruelty, and brutality" perpetuated on women of color and immigrants has continued in the form of persistent suspicion related to these women's use of birth control (Silliman, Fried, Ross, & Gutiérrez, 2016, p. 49). It is important to concede that the reasons for some people's wariness about birth control are complex and deeply rooted in our nation's history and that, in many cases, this wariness stems from racism and/or misogyny.

Despite current controversies and debates, almost all Americans continue to support birth control. In 2012, 90% of Americans, and 82% of U.S. Catholics, agreed that birth control is moral (Newport, 2012). According to the Guttmacher Institute (2018), 99% of Catholics and Protestants who have had sexual intercourse have ever used some form of contraception. In fact, among those at risk of unintended pregnancy, approximately 73% of Protestants and 74% of evangelicals use a highly effective method, such as hormonal contraception, sterilization, or an IUD. Although the vast majority of Americans favor unrestricted access to birth control, the issue remains an area of intense debate and disagreement. What has been described as an American culture war—those opposing the "war on religion" against those decrying a "war on women"—affects public policy at both the federal and state level.

What laws and regulations make it easier for women to access birth control?

Although many individuals and organizations consider birth control to be a global issue that transcends geographic borders, individual governments have their own laws, regulations, and policies. Policy has a significant effect on access to contraception, and birth control access and affordability can transform alongside political and governmental changes, even in developed countries such as the United States. According to Wyer, Barbercheck, Cookmeyer, Ozturk, and Wayne (2014), "the increasing visibility of women's health care in public policy discussions" over the past few decades is a sign of progress in women's health in the United States (p. xiv). Indeed, with mostly bipartisan support in the past 60 years, birth control has become safer, cheaper, and more accessible overall (Office of Women's Health, 2014).

Across the United States, numerous birth control laws and regulations at both the federal and state level have developed over decades. In 1959, President Dwight Eisenhower refused to discuss contraception, declaring, "I cannot imagine anything more emphatically a subject that is not a proper political or governmental activity or function or responsibility." However, by the 1960s and 1970s, federal U.S. policies and regulations that addressed contraception focused on access and cost. In 1969, Republican President, Richard Nixon famously said, "No American woman should be denied access to family planning assistance because of her economic condition." Just a year later, in 1970, the U.S. government passed Title X of the Public Service Act. This act established federally funded family planning centers to assist poorer women with contraception and family planning. It also provided noncontraceptive health-related services, including care for pregnant women, cancer screenings, and sexually transmitted infections testing. Today, Title X helps four million women a year access reproductive health care, and the clinics funded under Title X prevent approximately one million unintended pregnancies each year. Administered by the U.S. Department of Health and Human Services' Office of Population Affairs, Title X remains the only federally funded assistance program focused on birth control today. As we discuss later in this chapter, however, in the past few years, Title X has come under attack.

Particularly significant in terms of the laws and regulations on birth control was the ACA, implemented under the presidency of Barack Obama in 2012, which we discuss in detail in the next section. The ACA mandated that health insurance plans offer cost-free contraception to women, increasing access for millions of American women.

State laws and regulations on birth control vary widely across the United States. While some states in recent years have attempted to legislate to decrease access to contraception, others have pursued a different tactic. According to the Guttmacher Institute (2016), 28 states currently require their state health insurance plans to cover hormonal contraceptives. More specifically,

- 11 states require coverage of methods received over the counter; the insurer may still require the enrollee to obtain a prescription.
- 19 states and the District of Columbia require insurers to cover an extended supply of contraceptives at one time.
- 6 states require coverage of male sterilization, and 11 states require coverage of female sterilization. (Guttmacher Institute, 2016)

As of 2019, the following states have policies that provide free birth control to women:

- California
- Illinois
- Maine
- Maryland
- Massachusetts
- New York
- Nevada
- Oregon
- Vermont

Overall, however, it is impossible to generalize about state laws and policies on contraception; evidence demonstrates a wide range of legislation and policies across the United States at the state level.

How does the Affordable Care Act impact access to birth control?

One of the most significant developments in increasing access to birth control in the United States was the ACA, also known as "Obamacare." Passed in 2010 under the Obama administration and implemented in 2012, the ACA included a "Women's Health Amendment" designed to ensure that women would have access to essential services, including preventive care (cancer screenings, prenatal care, mammograms, etc.) at no cost to themselves. The ACA also required most health insurance plans in the United States to cover all methods of birth control approved by the U.S. Food and Drug Administration (FDA). Known as the "contraceptive mandate," this part of the ACA required companies and businesses with at least 50 employees to offer health insurance plans that would provide cost-free birth control to women. This mandate received enthusiastic support from some legislators. As Senator Kirsten Gillibrand said during the Senate debates on the ACA,

> [N]ot only do [women] pay more for the coverage we seek for the same age and the same coverage as men do, but in general women of childbearing age spend 68 percent more in out-of-pocket health care costs than men. . . . This fundamental inequity in the current system is dangerous and discriminatory and we must act. The prevention section of the bill before us must be amended so coverage of preventive services takes into account the unique health care needs of women throughout their life-span. (Lipton-Lubet, 2014, p. 347)

The ACA requires that employers' health insurance plans cover 18 FDA-approved methods of contraception free of cost, without charging copays or deductibles (Guttmacher Institute, 2016). The birth control methods covered under the ACA are

- Female sterilization surgery (tubal ligation).
- Implant.
- Copper IUD.
- Hormonal IUD.
- Shot/injection.
- Oral contraceptives.
- The patch.
- Vaginal contraceptive ring.
- Diaphragm.
- Sponge.
- Cervical cap.
- Female condom.
- Spermicide.
- Emergency contraception.

The effects of the ACA have been profound. Because of it, out-of-pocket birth control costs in the United States declined significantly (Snyder, Weisman, Liu, Leslie, & Chuang, 2018). With cost issues alleviated for many, more women used birth control, mostly hormonal methods. Significantly, the use of LARC methods increased in the wake of the contraceptive mandate. One study found a substantial increase in IUD use from 2011 to 2013 (Snyder et al., 2018). In 2013, the ACA helped women save an estimated $1.4 billion on the pill. Between October 2013 and March 2014, over four million women received health insurance coverage through the ACA. In the next section, we discuss opposition to the ACA and attempts to roll back the contraceptive mandate.

Some researchers and commentators have criticized the ACA's focus on women rather than all people. The contraceptive mandate, for example, does not cover the male condom or male sterilization (vasectomy). As the website bedsider.org notes, "this might not seem like a big deal, until you realize that almost 1 in 4 women (23%) rely on their partners' vasectomies or use of condoms as their main way to prevent pregnancy" ("Men's Health," 2018). The ACA's failure to cover male forms of birth control, some argue, reinforces the idea that fertility control is solely the responsibility of women, leaving men free from such responsibilities.

What laws and regulations make it difficult for women to access birth control?

As we discussed in Chapter 2, there is a complex legal history of birth control in United States. Changing political administrations have led to significant policy shifts on contraception since the late twentieth century. During the 1980s, for example, the Republican Reagan administration, informed by the New Right and evangelicalism, cut federal funding to Title X programs and initiatives by 25%. Then, with the subsequent election of the Democratic Bill Clinton in 1992, the pendulum shifted again. Clinton almost immediately raised spending for family planning, with Title X spending increasing by more than 37% in just a few years (Critchlow, 1999, pp. 103–104).

Laws and regulations have changed significantly in just the past few years as well. When the ACA was signed into law in 2010, it increased access to family planning for millions of Americans. After the ACA came into effect, however, some politicians, employers, and organizations protested its contraceptive mandate. Legal challenges to the ACA have been significant; over 80 lawsuits targeting the contraceptive mandate have gone forward. The most well-known of these occurred in 2014, when Hobby Lobby, a major employer that has hundreds of craft supply stores across the United States, challenged the ACA's directive to offer birth control to its employees. Citing the Religious Freedom Restoration Act of 1993, the owners of Hobby Lobby argued that, by forcing it to provide contraception to its employees, the ACA was infringing on the company's religious beliefs. As *Time* magazine summarized, "the company objected to paying for emergency contraception including Plan B, Ella—both commonly known as the morning after pill—plus two types of IUDs. Hobby Lobby said they believe these types of birth control amount to abortion" (Dockterman, 2014).

The case, *Burwell vs. Hobby Lobby*, eventually made its way to the U.S. Supreme Court. In June 2014, the Supreme Court ruled in favor of Hobby Lobby, writing that any employer "with deeply held religious beliefs" could, under law, "opt out" of covering birth control through its health insurance plans. The ruling effectively meant that the government could no longer require employers to provide insurance coverage for birth control if birth control was seen as conflicting with the employer's religious beliefs (Lipton-Lubet, 2014, p. 344). The 2014 Supreme Court decision stated that only closely held companies (companies in which five or fewer people own 50% of the company) could exempt themselves from the ACA's contraceptive mandate.

When Donald Trump became president, this changed. In early 2017, Trump said in a speech: "We will not allow people of faith to be targeted, bullied, or silenced anymore." In October 2017, the Trump administration's Justice Department instructed all American employers that they should feel free to exempt themselves from the contraceptive mandate "on the basis of religious objections." Simultaneously, the Department of Health and Human Services created new policies that removed the contraceptive mandate for *any* employer, not just closely held companies, if that employer had religious objections to doing so (Pear, Ruiz, & Goodstein, 2017). Thus far, federal appeals courts have blocked these rulings from being implemented, but as of late 2019, debates and legal maneuverings continue, with some experts predicting that the issue will end up at the Supreme Court.

The Trump administration also has acted to revise Title X. The so-called domestic gag rule (2019) prohibits Title X-funded organizations from providing abortion services or abortion referrals. As a result, some organizations will be forced to either stop providing abortion services and information or leave Title X. In fact, in August 2019, Planned Parenthood announced its intention to exit the Title X program because of the government's new guidelines. Currently, 40% of women who receive Title X services do so through Planned Parenthood (McCammon, 2019). According to the nonprofit independent news organization Common Dreams, "The loss of $60 million for Planned Parenthood means that 1.5 million low-income women—40 percent of the women across the country who obtain healthcare funded by Title X—could lose the medical care they receive at the group's clinics" (Conley, 2019).

Other laws and regulations in the United States also prevent people from accessing contraception. In recent years, emergency contraception (EC) has been subject to controversy and challenges. In addition to employer objections, like those highlighted in the 2014 Hobby Lobby case, pharmacists have cited conscience clauses to deny services. Some pharmacists oppose dispensing EC, claiming that their religious beliefs should exempt them from providing contraceptive services. In addition, some pharmacies refuse to even stock EC. A 2012 study found that some pharmacists who will not dispense EC have serious misconceptions about EC and believe myths about EC, including that it causes birth defects or can induce abortion (Richman et al., 2012). Currently, under law, six U.S. states (Arizona, Arkansas, Georgia, Idaho, Mississippi, and South Dakota) permit pharmacists to deny medications to clients based on religious objections ("conscience clauses"). Meanwhile, eight states (California, Illinois, Nevada, Maine, Massachusetts, New Jersey, Washington, and Wisconsin) "have laws explicitly prohibiting medication refusals" ("Pharmacists Refusing," 2018).

Is cost a barrier to consistent use of contraception?

Cost remains a significant barrier to consistent contraceptive use in the United States.

According to a 2012 study, women who had private insurance paid about half of the total cost of their birth control pills. For these women, the cost of the pill constitutes 29% of their out-of-pocket health-care costs. Women who need birth control spend, on average, 68% more on out-of-pocket health-care costs than do men of a similar age (Arons, 2012). As some employers and government officials successfully challenge both Title X and the ACA's contraceptive mandate, the costs of birth control for many women are increasing.

Millions of people, meanwhile, lack health insurance in the United States. For these people, affording birth control can be challenging. Condoms cost around $1 each. Most birth control pills, without insurance, cost approximately $20 to $50 per month. This adds up to between $240 and $600 per year. The shot costs between $200 to $300 per year. The patch costs about $1,200 per year, IUDs can cost more than $1,000, and the implant costs around $800. This means that the methods that experts recommend and consider to be most effective (LARC methods) are the most cost-prohibitive for many. People consider cost when choosing a contraceptive method; "among women aged 18–44 surveyed in 2016, more than 70% said that it was 'extremely or quite important' for their contraceptive method to be low cost" (Guttmacher Institute, 2016).

Women's words and narratives affirm their support for low-cost or free contraception. According to one woman, who received Depo-Provera® for free under Title X, "It's about 'being able to afford health care and how that can make a person whole, and thrive'" (Washington, 2019). Similarly, one of our interviewees linked inexpensive birth control to her overall economic status, saying that for her, access to affordable birth control provided "peace of mind. Not living in abject poverty for my whole life." Another narrator described the financial obstacles related to health insurance and how essential low-cost services were to her: "I was getting birth control out of the health department. Insurance didn't pay for it. If you went to the health department, they were free."

Does health insurance cover contraception?

Some health insurance providers in the United States are publicly funded; others are private. Public health insurance programs include Medicaid, Medicare, TRICARE, the Indian Health Service (IHS), and Title X funded clinics. Medicaid is a state-federal program that provides health coverage to individuals with low incomes. All Medicaid programs are required to cover family planning services and supplies. In 2011, at least 3.5 million women aged 15 to 49 obtained Medicaid-covered family planning services through family planning waivers (Kaiser Family Foundation, 2015). Although Medicare coverage is primarily for people over 65, about a million younger people with disabilities also qualify for Medicare, and some of these people need birth control ("Does Your Medicare Plan," n.d.).

People employed by the U.S. military and their dependents also need access to reliable and affordable contraception. Approximately 95% of American women serving in the military are of reproductive age. TRICARE, the federal military health-care program, provides most birth control free of cost for women on active military duty. Women not on active duty or women dependents of employees of the military must pay copays for contraception. For people on active duty stationed across the world, however, it is sometimes difficult to access birth control; different military health clinics may only have certain forms of contraception available (Grindlay, 2016). On military bases within the United States, approximately 50% to 88% of women use contraceptives regularly. On bases outside of the United States, however, that range decreases to 39% to 77%. Today, "inadequate contraceptive counseling and care before deployment—as well as lack of care and supplies while deployed—may contribute to increased rates of unintended pregnancy among servicewomen" (Rugg & Barry, 2015). The U.S. Department of Veterans Affairs (VA) also offers low-cost or cost-free methods of contraception for women veterans, and some VA medical centers "have a Women Veterans Program Manager to help women Veterans access VA benefits and health care services" (VA, n.d.).

The IHS (n.d.), a federal government division within the Department of Health and Human Services, has a mandate "to raise the physical, mental, social, and spiritual health of American Indians and Alaska Natives to the highest level." Currently, the IHS provides health care to over two million Americans. It offers contraception coverage as well, although access to contraceptives vary throughout particular IHS facilities. In June 2013, the FDA approved the EC progestin pill One-Step (Plan B) for sale in the United States over the counter for any person of any age. In response, IHS created a new policy stating: "It is IHS policy the Plan B One-Step® emergency contraception pill is easily available through the IHS facilities' pharmacy, Emergency Department (ED), and in health clinics that are equipped with secure medication storage areas" (IHS, 2015).

Some private health insurance plans in the United States cover contraception. This differs based on multiple factors, including which state a person lives in and who their employer is. The ACA created the first federal contraceptive coverage requirement for private plans, but as we discussed earlier, employers with religious or moral objections may opt out of the contraceptive mandate.

At the state level, policies and laws on insurance coverage differ. In April 1998, Maryland became the first state to mandate that insurance companies cover birth control. In the years following the ACA, eight states, including California and Massachusetts, expanded access to free contraception. In California, pharmacists can dispense oral contraceptive pills without a physician's prescription. In 2017, Oregon passed the Reproductive Health Equity Act, which ensures that women not only have access to free birth control, including vasectomies, but also provides for cost-free abortion. Significantly, the act extends these benefits to "women who are undocumented including DACA recipients and women who have held lawful permanent resident status for less than five years" (Oregon Health Authority, n.d.). When she signed the law, Governor Kate Brown said, "Everyone deserves the ability to make informed decisions about their health and to control their bodies, which shouldn't be dependent upon where they live, where they come from, or how they identify."

How does access to contraception vary in the United States, and what are its effects?

As we discussed in Chapter 1 of this book, equal access to contraception is necessary to achieve reproductive justice. Access to contraception, however, remains a serious barrier to consistent use. Today in the United States, a person's ability to use birth control consistently depends on various factors, including geography, socioeconomic position, and cultural issues. In a 2015 document, the American Public Health Association (APHA, 2015) noted:

> Both in the United States and globally, specific populations encounter greater barriers to contraception access than the general population. These underserved populations include residents of rural areas, adolescents (unmarried and married girls), minority and indigenous communities, groups living in conflict zones or in areas affected by natural disasters, refugees and migrants (especially undocumented migrants), people with mental or physical disabilities, people living in extreme poverty, girls and women in violent intimate relationships, women and girls living in societies where their mobility outside the home is restricted, employees of religious organizations that oppose contraception, and residents of areas where health services are overseen by such organizations.

Particularly troubling is the reality that almost 20 million American women today live in what are called "contraceptive deserts." This means that they lack reasonable access to birth control because of a lack of health centers or providers. Contraceptive deserts are areas where there is less than one health provider or clinic for every 1,000 women. Today, 1,570,720 women in the United States "live in counties without access to a single health center that provides the full range of methods" (Power to Decide, n.d.). Power to Decide estimates that 97% of women aged 13 to 44 who are in need of contraception currently live in contraceptive deserts.

Many people who live in contraceptive deserts are disadvantaged by other related factors as well, including race or ethnicity, sexuality, immigration status, and ability. A recent study concluded, for example, that

> although young African-American women tend to live closer to pharmacies than their white counterparts (1.2 miles to the nearest pharmacy for African Americans vs. 2.1 miles for whites), those pharmacies tend to be independent pharmacies (59 vs. 16%) that are open fewer hours per week (64.6 vs. 77.8) and have fewer female pharmacists (17 vs. 50%), fewer patient brochures on contraception (2 vs. 5%), more difficult access to condoms (49% vs. 85% on the shelf instead of behind glass, behind the counter, or not available), and fewer self-check-out options (3 vs. 9%). More African-American than white women live near African-American pharmacists (8 vs. 3%). These race differences are regardless of poverty, measured by the receipt of public assistance. (Barber et al., 2019, abstract.)

We must therefore put contraceptive access within a larger context, asking how and why accessing such essential health care remains difficult for so many and considering the intersecting factors that contribute to a lack of access to birth control.

Although many LGBTQ+ people need birth control, misconceptions and ignorance continue to prevent some from accessing it. LGBTQ+ individuals, including transgender men and nonbinary, queer, or bisexual people, can engage in sexual practices that may result in pregnancy. Yet scholarly research on LGBTQ+ access to contraception remains rare, and many health care providers remain ignorant about this population's contraceptive needs. As Neesha Powell (2017) writes, "when we talk about birth control, we need to remember that cis straight women aren't the only stakeholders. As a pansexual nonbinary woman, birth control changed my life for the

better, yet narratives like mine are missing from the media."
According to one resident of Texas in their 20s,

> I had a tubal ligation done about a year ago. I am a bi
> transmasculine person. Before I had the procedure, my
> fertility (the thought of being pregnant) was giving me
> reoccurring nightmares. I was limiting my sexual en-
> counters out of fear of pregnancy. I've never tried any
> other form of birth control besides condoms and my
> tubal ligation. After having the surgery I have so much
> less anxiety around sex. (Bell, 2019)

In addition, thousands of LGBTQ+ people use hormonal forms
of birth control for noncontraceptive reasons, including controlling menstruation and treating related conditions.

Another population that is often overlooked in studies of
birth control access is incarcerated women. Studies show that
providing incarcerated women with reliable birth control before they are released from prison can affect their subsequent
unintended pregnancy rates. Women given contraception
while in prison are much more likely to use it consistently
after their release. Moreover, women who enter prison and
may have had unprotected sex in the days before their incarceration need access to EC. According to one recent survey, almost 30% of recently incarcerated women had unprotected sex
in the days before entering prison. Some incarcerated women
also experience rape and sexual assault during their imprisonment; they, too, need access to EC, as do some incarcerated
women who are allowed conjugal visits. Despite these clear
needs, prison systems across the United States have a wide
variety of policies on providing EC to incarcerated women.
As of 2016, only 4% of facilities nationwide had EC on hand
(Driver, 2018).

In today's political and cultural climate, in which migrants,
refugees, and asylum-seekers have come under increased

scrutiny, more research needs to be done on what sort of access these groups have to contraception, both during and after their journeys to the United States. Immigrant women in general in the United States tend to have less access to health insurance and contraception, and refugees and asylum-seekers face additional access issues. According to the Women's Refugee Commission (n.d.), "Not being able to access family planning threatens [refugees'] lives and the well-being of their families."

Several news stories in 2019 hinted at the realities of reproductive experiences for some migrant women. According to Maylin Nuñez, a 17-year-old Honduran making the journey through Mexico to the United States, preparing for her trip included securing access to birth control. Nuñez, a married mother of one, received a birth control shot before leaving Honduras because she was not sure if she would be able to access contraception while in route. Undocumented women journeying to the United States also are vulnerable to sexual assault. According to Amnesty International, 80% of women migrants experience rape and sexual assault during their migration journeys. These women have little access to EC (Fleury, 2016).

Another vulnerable population that struggles to access birth control is homeless or housing-insecure women. Seventy-three percent of homeless Americans claim that they have health needs that are not being addressed or cared for. American College of Obstetricians and Gynecologists (ACOG, 2013) writes that

> women and families are the fastest growing segment of the homeless population, with 34% of the total homeless population composed of families. Of these homeless families, 84% are headed by women. African American families are disproportionately represented among the homeless population, making up 43% of homeless families.

A 2017 Chicago-based study revealed that "while 94% of the homeless women surveyed wanted to avoid pregnancy, most were using the least effective contraceptive methods. Among the women currently using a method, 59% relied on condoms, while 27% relied on withdrawal" (Corey, Frazin, Heywood, & Haider, 2017).

As we detail in the conclusion, telehealth initiatives and innovations promise to improve some vulnerable groups' access to birth control.

What role do regulatory bodies such as the FDA play in birth control?

The FDA is the United States' regulatory body for all forms of medical devices and drugs. It is responsible for approving forms of contraception and thus allowing them to be marketed and sold in the United States. In 1960, the FDA famously approved Enovid as the first oral contraceptive pill available for contraceptive use. Since 1960, the FDA has approved dozens of forms of birth control for use and consumption in the United States, including LARC methods. Some methods of contraception that are available in other parts of the world, however, have not received FDA approval and thus are not accessible by American women. In the United States, for example, only five types of IUDs are available. In Britain, however, 22 types of IUDs are available to women, and Canadian women have access to 9 kinds of IUDs, all with different shapes (Beaton, 2017). As we discussed in Chapter 2 of this volume, after the Dalkon Shield controversy in the 1970s, the FDA stepped in to regulate IUDs. It currently classifies them as drugs, subjecting them to longer approval processes.

In rare cases, the FDA also has removed approval from certain contraceptives. As we discussed in Chapter 1 of this volume, in 2018, the FDA restricted the sale and distribution of Essure®, an implantable device that leads to permanent sterilization in women. It consists of two "soft, flexible inserts" that, in a "gentle, non-surgical" procedure, are passed through the vagina and cervix into the fallopian tubes. There, the inserts, which do not contain or release hormones, help generate scar tissue that blocks the tubes. (Block, 2017)

In 2002, the FDA fast-tracked Essure® for approval. In the years following, thousands of women complained about harmful side effects and damaging consequences; approximately 9,000 American women ultimately had the device removed. These complications sparked serious criticism of the FDA. In 2015, researchers at Yale wrote,

We believe that these safety concerns, along with problems with the device's effectiveness, might have been detected sooner or avoided altogether if there had been higher-quality premarketing and postmarketing evaluations and more timely and transparent dissemination of study results. (Block, 2017)

The same year, after five women died from Essure® complications, the FDA began a review of the device. This review resulted in the FDA withdrawing its approval from Essure® in 2018.

In recent years, " 'femtech'—technology aimed at women's health, which analysts estimate will become a $50 billion market by 2025," has exploded in popularity (Lieber, 2018). As part of this phenomenon, "fertility awareness" apps, including Clue, Kindara, Ovia, and Glow, have become more common in the United States. These apps, which assist with natural family planning methods, feature cycle tracking tools. In 2018, the FDA caused some controversy when it approved one of these apps, Natural Cycles, as a form of contraception. Once a woman enters her menstrual cycle details and basal body temperature readings, the app informs the woman which days of the month she will be fertile. The FDA expedited the approval process for Natural Cycles and ultimately categorized it as a medical device. This, in turn, resulted in criticisms by some physicians and experts, who argue that natural family planning techniques are problematic and should not be categorized as contraception. As Lieber (2018) reported:

> Lauren Streicher, a professor of clinical obstetrics and gynecology at Northwestern University's Feinberg School of Medicine, said an app like Natural Cycles is "problematic on so many levels." She said the FDA's approval of the technology left her infuriated and speechless. "This isn't science; this is craziness," Streicher said. "We've already developed good, safe, reliable methods of contraception that are available to us. This app is completely taking women back in time."

What education about birth control is available today?

In 1912, American social worker and reformer Jane Addams wrote: "The child growing up in the midst of civilization receives from its parents and teachers something of the accumulated experience of the world on all other subjects save upon that of sex" (Addams 1912). In the early twentieth century, Addams and other reformers began to advocate for sex education in public schools. Linked to the growth of the federal government, the public school revolution, and the popularity of hygiene movements, sex education increased across the country (Zimmerman, 2015). By the postwar era, new technologies were enhancing the options for sex education. Educational films in the late 1940s and 1950s, for example, became ubiquitous learning tools for many American students. Although sex education in public schools in the mid-twentieth century did not offer comprehensive information on birth control, this changed by the 1970s and 80s, when evidence suggesting that adolescents were increasingly sexually active combined with the AIDS crisis to create a sense of urgency (Ashbee, 2014, p. 102).

Here, again, however, we see shifts in practices because of larger political changes. In the 1980s, the rise of the New Right and the evangelical purity movement began to have effects on sex education. Abstinence-only education teaches that no sex before marriage should be the norm. These programs generally do not teach about birth control or sexually transmitted infections. So-called abstinence-only programs became more common in the 1980s and 1990s, and increasingly received not only greater federal support but also funding. Meanwhile, support for contraceptive education declined. When George W. Bush became president in 2001, he increased funding for abstinence-only education. In the years since, abstinence-only education continues to dominate in the United States.

Studies and surveys by the Centers for Disease Control and Prevention and others have shown that almost all American adolescents—approximately 95%—receive some sort of sex education. From 2006 to 2013, however, as data from the National Survey of Family Growth demonstrated, teenagers' knowledge of, and education about, contraception declined sharply. According to Planned Parenthood: "21% of females and 35% of males report not receiving information about birth control from either formal sources or their parents" ("Planned Parenthood | Official Site," n.d.).

Women we interviewed in the past decade almost uniformly expressed a lack of education about contraception throughout their childhoods and adolescences, both at home and at school. A major theme around birth control in childhood was silence. One participant discussed how "contraception is . . . not something that was talked about often either because that meant you were having sex." Another told us about sex in general: "My parents never really, they were just kind of like don't do it. So honestly I was a little bit in the dark.

I wasn't reading magazines at the time that would have maybe put things into layman's terms for me." Another said, "My father, I remember being in elementary school, and he wouldn't even let us see cats being born on TV. And I lived on a farm but I had no idea what was going on." Our participants also clearly linked a lack of early education about birth control to later practices. One participant noted, "But for somebody in my demographic, that's a woman, who comes from a place that—we didn't really have means . . . your options are limited, and when you don't know any better, you can't do any better."

Today, regional variations in funding and educational content, abstinence-only education in many public schools, a continued reluctance by parents and guardians to discuss a full range of options, and lack of physician education and knowledge about birth control all contribute to a persistent and troubling ignorance about contraception.

What is the status of birth control in the United States today?

As this chapter has demonstrated, policies relating to birth control are always shifting. As of late 2019, this pattern continues. So do debates and controversies. Currently in focus are the Trump administration's changes to the Title X program, continued divisions over abortion, and legal wrangling associated with the contraceptive mandate. According to the Guttmacher Institute,

> reproductive health programs and key providers of reproductive health care are under siege in the United States. Social conservatives in Congress are attempting to wipe out funding for the Title X national family planning program, negate the guarantee of contraceptive coverage under the Affordable Care Act (ACA) and defund Planned Parenthood at the national and state levels. (Barot, 2015)

A recent poll conducted by the Kaiser Family Foundation (2019a) revealed that a majority of American women "are concerned that access to women's reproductive health and preventive care services may be limited by the Trump administration's changes to Title X, the nation's federal family planning program."

Still, the most prominent scientific, medical, and public health associations support unrestricted access to cost-free contraception. The ACOG (n.d.), which is the main professional organization for obstetricians and gynecologists in the United States, for example, notes: "Ob-gyns, physicians whose primary responsibility is women's health, are dedicated to providing scientific information and access to contraception for their patients." The APHA (n.d.), according to its website,

champions the health of all people and all communities. We strengthen the public health profession. We speak out for public health issues and policies backed by science. We are the only organization that combines a nearly 150-year perspective, a broad-based member community and the ability to influence federal policy to improve the public's health.

In 2015, the APHA (2015) affirmed its support for birth control, stating:

This policy supports the universal right to contraception access in the United States and internationally. Contraceptive use confers significant health benefits through reductions in unwanted and high-risk pregnancies, maternal and infant morbidity and mortality, unsafe abortions, and medical therapy. These benefits are so significant that universal access to contraception is accepted internationally as essential to human rights.

These organizations recognize the importance of contraceptive access and advocate for continued education, resources, and support for birth control. Similarly, our interviewees articulated not only their support for birth control but their awareness that in the United States today, access remains problematic. As one said, "I think we've come a far way, you know, I think there's a lot more work to be done."

What are global or transnational policies on birth control?

In 1994, the United Nations (UN) Population Fund declared reproductive rights, including universal access to contraception, to be fundamental human rights. At the same time, the UN "also identified four 'interrelated and essential' principles that constitute the right to the highest attainable standard of health: availability, accessibility, acceptability, and quality" (APHA, 2015). In the years since, the international community has overwhelmingly affirmed its support for birth control access and education.

Improving access to family planning services can help lower unintended pregnancy rates and reduce maternal deaths. According to the Kaiser Family Foundation, "Each year, an estimated 303,000 women die from complications during pregnancy and childbirth. . . . Approximately one-third of maternal deaths could be prevented annually if women who did not wish to become pregnant had access to and used effective contraception" (Kaiser Family Foundation, 2019b). Today across the world, however, around 214 million women who need or want contraception are not able to access it and/or afford it (Guttmacher Institute, 2016).

International health-focused organizations have been working for decades to increase birth control education, affordability, and access across the globe. These organizations are generally divided into three groups: multilateral organizations, bilateral organizations, and nongovernmental organizations (NGOs). Multilateral organizations are formed by multiple nations (usually at least three) to explore certain issues affecting the global community. The UN, WHO, and World Bank are examples of multilateral organizations working on global health care. Bilateral organizations may be linked with or sponsored by a particular government or may be NGOs. They are usually based in one country but conduct research about and work in areas other than their home country. The Centers for Disease Control and Prevention and U.S. Agency for International Development (USAID) are two bilateral organizations working on global health care. NGOs are nonprofit organizations, not linked with any particular government, that address particular transnational issues including health care. Health-care focused examples include Doctors Without Borders and the Kaiser Family Foundation (Center for Global Health, n.d.).

The previously mentioned international health-based organizations consistently advocate for birth control access and availability in our world today. Indeed, there is a consensus among these organizations that birth control is a fundamental right and that all people, across national borders, should have affordable access to it. The UN Family Planning Association (UNFPA) is the UN's sexual and reproductive health unit. It publishes information and research that can help different governments and NGOs develop policies about birth control. The UNFPA (n.d.) "calls for the realization of reproductive rights for all and supports access to a wide range of sexual and reproductive health services—including voluntary family planning, maternal health care and comprehensive sexuality education." It argues that "access to safe, voluntary family planning is a human right. Family planning is central to gender equality and women's empowerment, and it is a key factor in reducing poverty" (UNFPA, n.d.). Similarly, the WHO (2018) argues, "Promotion of family planning—and ensuring access to preferred contraceptive methods for women and couples—is essential to securing the well-being and autonomy of women, while supporting the health and development of communities."

Despite the consensus among NGOs, multilateral organizations, and bilateral organizations that birth control is essential in the twenty-first century, actually implementing policies to facilitate greater access and education can be difficult. This is complicated in different parts of the world by various factors. As the WHO summarizes, people in developing countries sometimes confront the following obstacles:

- limited choice of methods;
- limited access to contraception, particularly among young people, poorer segments of populations, or unmarried people;
- fear or experience of side effects;
- cultural or religious opposition;
- poor quality of available services;
- users and providers bias; and
- gender-based barriers. (WHO, 2013)

As this chapter has outlined, however, the challenges and obstacles are not limited to the developing world. In the United States, various factors, including lack of knowledge/education, restrictive legislative measures, and prohibitive cost prevent some people from accessing contraception.

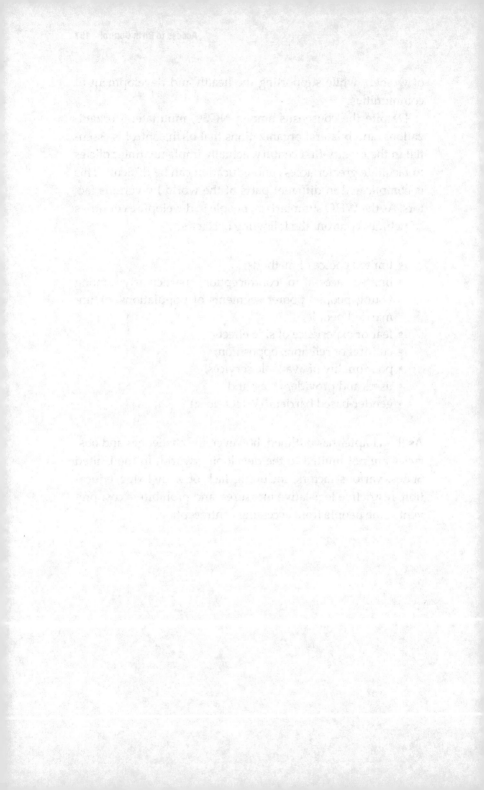

CONCLUSION

WHAT IS THE FUTURE OF
BIRTH CONTROL?

Beyond women?

As we have discussed in this book, an analysis of birth control encourages us to privilege the experiences and voices of women. It also, however, suggests that we need to move beyond viewing birth control as something exclusively for women. Researchers have called for an expanded investigation of men and birth control. They argue that in the United States today, "pregnancy prevention programs that target young women overlook the pivotal role that young men can play in preventing unintended pregnancies" (Parekh, Finocharo, Kim, & Manlove, 2019, p. 48). Discussions of the future of men's roles in birth control have focused primarily on the creation of a hormonal birth control pill for men. Studies have shown that many men—over 55% in a recent study—"want to try new, hormonal male contraceptive methods if they are reversible" ("Male Birth Control," 2019). Scientists working on this have developed a pill that contains progestin and testosterone, which decreases or stops a man's sperm production. In 2019, one of these male birth control pills passed safety tests; it is therefore possible that a male pill will be available in the United States within several years. However, trials have also found that the common side effects of male hormonal contraception, such as acne, altered libido, night sweats, increased weight, and mood changes, may be unacceptable to many men. Experts caution that despite the success of efficacy and feasibility studies, commercialization and a marketable product approved for clinical use may not yet be on the horizon (Gava & Meriggiola, 2019).

As we have argued in this book, moving "beyond women" when discussing birth control also involves recognizing the contraceptive requirements of people across the gender spectrum. A person's need for birth control is not related to their gender identity but rather their health, sexual practices, and behaviors. Transgender adolescent men, in fact, have the same rates of unintended pregnancy as their cisgender peers. They also need and want birth control. In a recent study, 65% of transgender men "reported using at least one method of birth control either for contraception or for menstrual control" (Light, Wang, & Gomez-Lobo, 2017, p. 274). We need to devote more resources to studying the birth control needs of the LGBTQ+ community and educating physicians and other health care providers about the contraceptive needs of all people.

How is telehealth changing access to birth control?

Telehealth utilizes modern technology to increase people's access to health-care services. It allows medical professionals to diagnose and treat patients remotely. According to the Center for Connected Health Policy (n.d.), "telehealth is a collection of means or methods for enhancing health care, public health and health education delivery and support using telecommunications technologies." Examples of telehealth services include

- mobile health apps;
- live patient–doctor videoconferencing; and
- remote patient monitoring.

For people who face obstacles visiting a health-care provider in person, telehealth can be essential (Sundstrom, DeMaria,

Ferrara, Meier, & Billings, 2019). Some of the reasons why people find it difficult to travel to doctors' offices and clinics include work commitments, child care, lack of transportation, or long distance to a health-care facility.

Birth control is a health-care issue that is well-suited to telehealth initiatives. Because contraception is something that a majority of people who can become pregnant use in their lifetime, it is essential that people be able to access it. Access to contraception, however, is sporadic for many people, particularly in rural areas. Telehealth may help address barriers to contraceptive access for millions of Americans. In 2018, for example, a University of Chicago pilot program established a successful mobile health unit. It was able to treat "123 adolescents, predominately African-American and Latino and between the ages of 14 and 21" and offer services from "supplying [emergency contraceptives] to reproductive health counseling" (mHealthIntelligence, 2018).

Online telehealth apps are promising to increase access to birth control for certain vulnerable populations, including homeless women and sex workers. Popular apps that offer contraception include Lemonaid, Nurx, and Virtuwell. The Planned Parenthood Direct app is also available in select states and offers prescriptions for birth control pills. Other digital platforms include 28H-TwentyeightHealth, HeyDoctor, Pandia Health, PRJKT RUBY, and Simple Health. Not all of these options are available in all states. Generally, people who use these apps begin by answering several health-related questions through the app. In some cases, a videoconference with a health-care professional follows, and that professional, if appropriate, will prescribe contraception to the user. In other cases, no videoconference is necessary; instead, the physician prescribes the birth control after looking over the user's answers to the questionnaire. Once prescribed, the medicine is sent to the patient or to a local pharmacy. Some apps also offer cost-effective or free contraception. Nurx and Lemonaid, for example, only charge $15 per month for the oral contraceptive pill (OCP) even for people without health insurance coverage (West, 2018). Emergency contraception is also available through some apps. Nurx offers both Ella® and Plan B®. Studies have shown that birth control apps are particularly popular with people who live in contraceptive deserts. They also help people with limited mobility gain access to birth control. Even today, decades after the Americans With Disabilities Act (1990), thousands of people who need and want access to birth control are unable to get it. Women with disabilities face stark disparities in gaining access to reproductive health care, and telehealth promises to increase this access (Health Resources and Services Administration, 2017).

Despite the promise of telehealth, there are problems associated with it. Its success relies on reliable internet access and infrastructure, which do not exist in some areas. Digital security is also a concern in an era when many feel anxious about sharing personal health details over the Internet or through an app. Some states currently do not allow for purchasing birth control via telehealth apps. Furthermore, some insurance providers, including Medicare and Medicaid, do not offer full reimbursement or coverage of telehealth services ("What Is Telehealth?" 2018).

Can I get birth control online?

Online birth control prescriptions are available in certain states. Through the website and app Nurx, for example, people can enter information that a physician will review. The physician may issue a prescription, and, if so, birth control is shipped to the user, usually arriving within a few days. Although several contraceptive methods are available through online providers including Nurx, Lemonaid, Hers, and the Pill Club, most focus on providing women with the OCP. Emergency contraception, as we discussed earlier, can also be purchased online via certain websites or apps.

Why do experts want to move oral contraceptives over the counter?

In June 2019, Democratic representative Alexandria Ocasio-Cortez tweeted: "Psst! Birth control should be over-the-counter, pass it on." In a surprising move, Republican senator Ted Cruz responded: "I agree. Perhaps, in addition to the legislation we are already working on together to ban Members of Congress from becoming lobbyists, we can team up here as well. A simple, clean bill making birth control available over the counter (OTC). Interested?" This exchange reflects an important reality: in the past few years, efforts to make the birth control pill available OTC in the United States have gained widespread support. Moving oral contraceptives OTC (OCs OTC) has the potential to provide women greater access to the pill and to ensure that they use contraception without interruption. It therefore is an important tool in preventing unintended pregnancies in the United States.

Experts and clinicians agree that OCPs should be available OTC. Today in the United States, the pill remains the most popular form of contraception used by women. Yet for many, barriers to accessing the pill remain. Lack of insurance coverage and high cost sometimes combine with difficulties getting to a physician and therefore problems receiving a prescription for the pill. Moreover, stigma, embarrassment, and clinician refusal based on religious reasons can prevent some from accessing a prescription for OCPs. For sex workers and homeless women, seeing a physician for a prescription can be difficult and traumatic. According to the Guttmacher Institute (2015), moving OCs OTC would help alleviate many of these issues, "especially among women who are uninsured and those who lack the time, would need to arrange for child care or otherwise would find it difficult to visit a health care provider to obtain a prescription." While many people believe that they must visit a physician and be examined before receiving contraception, this is an outdated view. The World

Health Organization argues that doctors' visits, pelvic examinations, and screenings for sexually transmitted infections are not necessary for a birth control prescription. Other organizations and experts agree (American College of Obstetricians and Gynecologists, 2019; Curtis, Tepper, Jamieson, & Marchbanks, 2013; Grossman, 2015).

Is it safe?

As we discussed in Chapter 3 of this book, decades of research show that hormonal contraception is safe for women. Experts believe that birth control pills are probably safer than other medicines available OTC, such as Tylenol® and Advil®. Misconceptions persist, however. Many women erroneously believe that they must receive an in-person gynecological exam and contraceptive counseling before receiving the OCP and worry that if they do not, they may be vulnerable to increased side effects, improper usage, or decreased efficacy. This is not true, however, and moving OCs OTC is perfectly safe. Research shows that women are adept at self-screening for possible health conditions and can use a checklist to determine if the pill is appropriate for them.

Most experts recommend that the pill be available OTC, in fact, because it is such a safe medication (American College of Obstetricians and Gynecologists, 2012; Kaunitz, 2008). Progestin-only pills, in particular, have few side effects and are excellent candidates for OTC consumption. According to the OCs OTC Working Group (n.d.), which has been in operation since 2004,

> Making the pill available OTC would make it easier for women to access it, and could save them time and money. In addition to appointment costs, there can also be other costs related to a clinic visit, like for travel and

child care. Moving a pill over the counter could also keep women from having gaps in their birth control use since they wouldn't need to schedule a medical visit to get or refill a prescription.

In fact, the pill is already available OTC in over 100 countries worldwide, including Mexico, India, and China, and data from these places reveals that moving OCs OTC does not compromise health or safety in any way.

Would it still be covered by health insurance?

OTC birth control pills would be covered by health insurance in the same ways that prescription pills are covered. So as of right now, under the ACA, OCs OTC would be covered by a majority of American companies' health insurance plans. In 2019, Senator Murray (D-WA) and Representative Pressley (D-MA) introduced the Affordability Is Access Act, which would ensure that insurance companies cover OCs OTC without a prescription or copay.

Are there any campaigns that provide more information about OCs OTC?

Despite experts' support for OCs OTC, many people who can become pregnant are not aware of the movement. The purpose of the OCs OTC Working Group (n.d.), based at Ibis Reproductive Health, is, in part, to "initiate dialogue with health professions associations as well as organizations representing diverse groups of women and create informational materials appropriate for different audiences." The Free the Pill (n.d.) campaign uses Facebook, Twitter, and Instagram to advocate for OCs OTC and to disseminate current information about efforts to move the pill OTC.

How can I weigh the evidence to make the best birth control choice for me?

Each person has the right to make their own decision about what birth control option may be best for them. Ideally, these decisions are made by individuals in consultation with others, including medical professionals. Patient counseling for contraception, however, remains incomplete and problematic in some areas. In the studies we conducted over several years, women told us that they often consult partners, friends, and family when gathering information to make decisions about birth control. In addition, research done in books or online can be helpful in collecting information about birth control methods. The "femtech" industry, comprised of software, apps, and services that use technology to inform about women's health care, has changed how women receive information about birth control. "Ditching the taboos around female health and sexuality," these "companies are at the forefront of change and speak to the most urgent needs of women" (Alley, n.d.). Of course, consumers must be careful and cautious about the information they receive online. Research is necessary to determine reliable, scientific evidence and information. At the end of this conclusion, and throughout this book, we list several useful resources that may help people who can become pregnant make decisions about birth control.

When considering different birth control options, the following questions may also serve as a helpful guide:

1. Do I want to become pregnant in the next year?
2. What are my short-term and long-term family planning goals?
3. Do I want to have a period?
4. Do I have heavy menstrual bleeding?
5. Does my period negatively impact my daily life, such as going to school, work, or spending time with my family and friends?

6. Do I have particular beliefs or traditions that affect my choice of birth control?
7. Do I need or want my birth control to be reversible?
8. How important are contraceptive side-effects to me when considering a birth control option?
9. Do I need or want to consult with my sexual partner(s) and consider their desires or opinions before selecting a method?
10. Do I need or desire dual protection in my birth control method?
11. Do I want my birth control to also serve as a lifestyle drug by providing non-contraceptive benefits (e.g., treatment or regulation of irregular, heavy, or painful periods; treatment of acne, anemia, endometriosis, premenstrual syndrome, or premenstrual dysphoric disorder)?
12. How active do I want to be, or am I able to be, every day in terms of using birth control? How long do I want my birth control to last?
13. How accessible must my birth control method be?
14. How much money am I able or willing to spend on birth control? What are the best financially sound options for me?
15. Am I able to visit a physician in person, or might Telehealth be a good option for me?

Resources: How can I find more information?

The following online resources can help you find more information about birth control:

The American College of Obstetricians and Gynecologists (ACOG): acog.org
American Public Health Association (APHA): apha.org
Bedsider: bedsider.org
Centers for Disease Control and Prevention: cdc.org

Free the Pill: freethepill.org
Planned Parenthood: plannedparenthood.org
Power to Decide: powertodecide.org
United Nations Family Planning Association: unfpa.org
World Health Organization: who.int

REFERENCES AND FURTHER READING

Introduction

Berger, M. T., & Guidroz, K. (2010). *The intersectional approach: Transforming the academy through race, class, and gender.* Chapel Hill, NC: University of North Carolina Press.

Crenshaw, K. (1989). Demarginalizing the intersection of race and sex: A Black feminist critique of antidiscrimination doctrine, feminist theory and antiracist politics. *University of Chicago Legal Forum, 140,* 139–168.

hooks, b. (1984). *Feminist theory: From margin to center.* Cambridge, MA: South End Press.

Roberts, D. (1997). *Killing the Black body: Race, reproduction, and the meaning of liberty.* New York, NY: Vintage Books.

Ross, L., & Solinger, R. (2017). *Reproductive justice: An introduction* (1st ed.). Oakland, CA: University of California Press.

Sharf, B., & Vanderford, M. L. (2008). Illness narratives and social construction of health. In T. L. Thompson, R. Parrott, & J. F. Nussbaum (Eds.), *Handbook of health communication* (pp. 9–34). New York, NY: Routledge.

SisterSong. (2018). Reproductive justice. Retrieved from http://sistersong.net/reproductive-justice/

Solinger, R. (2016). Reproductive justice 101. *Signs: Journal of Women in Culture and Society, 41*(4), 986–987. doi:10.1086/685792

Sundstrom, B. L. (2015). *Reproductive justice and women's voices: Health communication across the lifespan.* Lanham, MD: Lexington Books.

Chapter 1

Akgul, S., Bonny, A. E., Ford, N., Holland-Hall, C., & Chelvakumar, G. (2019). Experiences of gender minority youth with the intrauterine system. *Journal of Adolescent Health, 65*(1), 32–38. doi:10.1016/j.jadohealth.2018.11.010

American College of Obstetricians and Gynecologists. (2015). Committee opinion no. 642 summary: Increasing access to contraceptive implants and intrauterine devices to reduce unintended pregnancy. *Obstetrics & Gynecology, 126*(4), 912. doi:10.1097/aog.0000000000001102

Aztlan-James, E. A., McLemore, M., & Taylor, D. (2017). Multiple unintended pregnancies in U.S. women: A systematic review. *Women's Health Issues, 27*(4), 407–413. doi:10.1016/j.whi.2017.02.002

Bahr, A. (2012, August 29). As memories of Dalkon Shield fade, women embrace IUDs again. *Ms.* Retrieved from https://msmagazine.com/2012/08/29/as-memories-of-dalkon-shield-fade-women-embrace-iuds-again/

Becker, B. J., & Betstadt, S. J. (2013). *Patient perception of safety of hormonal contraception compared to pregnancy.* Presented at the 61st Annual Clinical Meeting of the American College of Obstetricians and Gynecologists, New Orleans, LA.

Boonstra, H., Duran, V., Gamble, V. N., Blumenthal, P., Dominguez, L., & Pies, C. (2000). The "boom and bust phenomenon": The hopes, dreams, and broken promises of the contraceptive revolution. *Contraception, 61*(1), 9–25.

Centers for Disease Control and Prevention. (1999). Achievements in public health, 1900–1999: Family planning. *Morbidity and Mortality Weekly Reports, 48*(47), 1073–1080. https://www.cdc.gov/mmwr/preview/mmwrhtml/mm4847a1.htm

Djerassi, C. (1989). The bitter pill. *Science, 245*(4916), 356–361.

FP 2020. (2019). Rights-based family planning: Developing and implementing programs that aim to fulfill the rights of all individuals. Family Planning 2020. United Nations Foundation, Washington, DC. Retrieved from https://www.familyplanning2020.org/rightsinfp

Frost, J. J., & Lindberg, L. D. (2013). Reasons for using contraception: Perspectives of U.S. women seeking care at specialized family planning clinics. *Contraception, 87*(4), 465–472. doi:10.1016/j.contraception.2012.08.012

Gipson, J. D., Koenig, M. A., & Hindin, M. J. (2008). The effects of unintended pregnancy on infant, child, and parental health: A review of the literature. *Studies in Family Planning, 39*(1), 18–38.

Guttmacher Institute. (2013). Births Resulting from Unintended Pregnancies Cost Federal and State Governments $12.5 Billion in 2008. Retrieved from https://www.guttmacher.org/news-release/ 2013/births-resulting-unintended-pregnancies-cost-federal-and-state-governments-125.

Guttmacher Institute. (2014). Contraceptive use in the United States. Retrieved from http://www.guttmacher.org/pubs/fb_contr_use. html#2

Guttmacher Institute. (2016). Beyond birth control: The overlooked benefits of oral contraceptive pills. Retrieved from https://www.guttmacher.org/report/ beyond-birth-control-overlooked-benefits-oral-contraceptive-pills

Jensen, J. T., & Trussell, J. (2012). Communicating risk: Does scientific debate compromise safety? *Contraception, 86*(4), 327–329. doi:10.1016/j.contraception.2012.06.010

Jiménez, L., Johnson, K., & Page, C. (2017). Beyond the trees: Stories and strategies of environmental and reproductive justice. In: L. J. Ross, L. Roberts, E. Derkas, W. Peoples, & P. B. Toure (Eds.), *Radical reproductive justice: Foundations, theory, practice, critique* (pp. 361–380). New York: Feminist Press at CUNY.

Kaye, K., Gootman, J. A., Ng, A. S., & Finley, C. (2014). The benefits of birth control in America: Getting the facts straight. *The National Campaign to Prevent Teen and Unplanned Pregnancy*. Retrieved from https://powertodecide.org/what-we-do/information/resource-library/benefits-of-birth-control-in-america

Lindheim, S. R., Madeira, J. L., Bagavath, B., & Petrozza, J. C. (2019). Social media and Essure hysteroscopic sterilization: A perfect storm. *Fertility and Sterility, 111*(6), 1105–1106.

Maas, M. K., & Lefkowitz, E. S. (2015). Sexual esteem in emerging adulthood: Associations with sexual behavior, contraception use, and romantic relationships. *Journal of Sex Research, 52*(7), 795–806. doi:10.1080/00224499.2014.945112.

Mosher, W. D., Jones, J., & Abma, J. C. (2012). Intended and unintended births in the United States: 1982–2010. *National Health Statistics Reports, 55*, 1–28.

Parry, M. (2013). *Broadcasting birth control: Mass media and family planning*. New Brunswick, NJ: Rutgers University Press.

Power to Decide. (2018, November 3). New polling shows strong support for birth control as a basic part of women's health care. Retrieved from https://powertodecide.org/about-us/newsroom/new-polling-shows-strong-support-for-birth-control-basic-part-womens-health-care

Price, K. (2010). What is reproductive justice?: How women of color activists are redefining the pro-choice paradigm. *Meridians, 10*(2), 42–65.

Roberts, D. (1997). *Killing the Black body: Race, reproduction, and the meaning of liberty.* New York, NY: Pantheon Books.

Ross, L., Derkas, E., Peoples, W., Roberts, L., & Bridgewater, P. (2017). *Radical reproductive justice: Foundation, theory, practice, critique.* New York, NY: The Feminist Press.

Ross, L., & Solinger, R. (2017). *Reproductive justice: An introduction.* Oakland, CA: University of California Press.

Silliman, J. M., Fried, M. G., Ross, L., & Gutiérrez, E. R. (2016). *Undivided rights: Women of color organizing for reproductive justice.* Chicago, IL: Haymarket Books.

SisterSong. (n.d.). Reproductive justice. Retrieved from https://www.sistersong.net/reproductive-justice

Sundstrom, B. (2015). *Reproductive justice and women's voices: Health communication across the lifespan.* Lanham, MD: Lexington Books.

United Nations Population Fund. (n.d.). [Homepage]. Retrieved from https://www.unfpa.org/

Watkins, E. S. (2012). How the pill became a lifestyle drug: The pharmaceutical industry and birth control in the United States since 1960. *American Journal of Public Health, 102*(8), 1462–1472.

Chapter 2

19th century artifacts. (n.d.). *Dittrick Medical History Center.* Retrieved from https://artsci.case.edu/dittrick/online-exhibits/history-of-birth-control/contraception-in-america-1800-1900/19th-century-artifacts/

Collins, G. (2009). *When Everything Changed: The Amazing Journey of American Women from 1960 to the Present.* New York, NY: Little, Brown and Company.

Ferranti, M. (2009). From birth control to that "fresh feeling": A historical perspective on feminine hygiene in medicine and media. *Women & Health, 49*(8), 592–607.

Foley, D. (1999). Organizing for social change and policy reform: Lessons from the International Planned Parenthood Federation. *International Journal of Organization Theory & Behavior,* 2(1/2), 89–106.

Gazit, C. (Dir., Writer). (2003, February 24). The pill [transcript] (C. Gazit, D. Steward, H. Klotz, Prods.). *PBS.* Retrieved from https://www.pbs.org/wgbh/americanexperience/films/pill/#transcript

Gold, R. B. (2014). Guarding against coercion while ensuring access: A delicate balance. *Guttmacher Institute.* Retrieved from http://www.guttmacher.org/pubs/gpr/17/3/gpr170308.html

Guttmacher Institute. (2018). Contraceptive use in the United States. Retrieved from https://www.guttmacher.org/fact-sheet/contraceptive-use-united-states

Knowlton, C. (1832). Fruits of philosophy: A treatise on the population question. *Project Gutenberg.* Retrieved from http://www.gutenberg.org/files/38185/38185-h/38185-h.htm#link2HCH0003

Langham, W. (1597). *The Garden of Health: Conteyning the Sundry Rare and Hidden Vertues and Properties of All Kindes of Simples and Plants, Together with the Maner how They are to be Vsed and Applyed in Medicine for the Health of Mans Body, Against Diuers Diseases and Infirmities Most Common Amongst Men. Gathered by the Long Experience and Industrie of William Langham, Practitioner in Phisicke.* London, England: By the deputies of Christopher Barker.

Lieberman, H. (2017, June 8). A short history of the condom. *JSTOR Daily.* Retrieved from https://daily.jstor.org/short-history-of-the-condom/

McLaren, A. (1992). *A history of contraception: From antiquity to the present.* Oxford, England: Blackwell.

Meier, S., Sundstrom, B., & DeMaria, A. L. (2015, October). *Beyond a legacy of coercion: Long-acting reversible contraception (LARC) and social justice.* Presented at the American Public Health Association (APHA) Annual Meeting and Exposition: Socialist Caucus, Chicago, IL.

Morgan, J. L. (2004). *Laboring Women: Reproduction and Gender in New World Slavery.* Early American Studies Philadelphia: University of Pennsylvania Press.

Payne, J. B., Sundstrom, B., & DeMaria, A. L. (2016). A qualitative study of young women's beliefs about intrauterine devices: Fear of infertility. *Journal of Midwifery & Women's Health,* 61(4), 482–488. doi:10.1111/jmwh.12425

Riddle, J. M. (1992). *Contraception and abortion from the ancient world to the Renaissance*. Cambridge, MA: Harvard University Press.

Riddle, J. M. (1997). *Eve's herbs: A history of contraception and abortion in the West*. Cambridge, MA: Harvard University Press.

Rovner, J. (2013, February 21). Morning-after pills don't cause abortion, studies say [audio file]. *NPR: All Things Considered*. Retrieved from https://www.npr.org/sections/health-shots/2013/02/22/172595689/morning-after-pills-dont-cause-abortion-studies-say

Ruggiero, G. (1989). *The boundaries of Eros: Sex crime and sexuality in Renaissance Venice*. New York, NY: Oxford University Press.

Schoen, J. (2005). *Choice and coercion: Birth control, sterilization, and abortion in public health and welfare*. Chapel Hill, NC: University of North Carolina Press.

Schwartz, M. J. (2006). *Birthing a Slave: Motherhood and medicine in the antebellum South*. Cambridge, MA: Harvard University Press.

Smith, D. S. (1973). Family limitation, sexual control and domestic feminism in Victorian America. *Feminist Studies, 1*(3–4), 40–57.

Strulik, H., & Vollmer, S. (2015). The fertility transition around the world. *Journal of Population Economics, 28*(1), 31–44.

Sundstrom, B. (2015). *Reproductive justice and women's voices: Health communication across the lifespan*. Lanham, MD: Lexington Books.

Tone, A. (1997). Contraceptive consumers: Gender and the political economy of birth control in the 1930s. In Andrea Tone (Ed.), *Controlling reproduction: An American history* (pp. 211–232). Wilmington, DE: SR Books.

Tone, A. (2001). *Devices and desires: A history of contraceptives in America* (1st ed). New York, NY: Hill and Wang.

Upadhyay, U. D. (2005). New Contraceptive Choices. Population Reports No. 19. Series M. Baltimore, MD: The Johns Hopkins Bloomberg School of Public Health.

Watkins, E. S. (2012). How the pill became a lifestyle drug: The pharmaceutical industry and birth control in the United States since 1960. *American Journal of Public Health, 102*(8), 1462–1472. doi:10.2105/AJPH.2012.300706

Wheaton, R. (1980). *Family and sexuality in French history*. University of Pennsylvania Press.

Wilkie, L. (2013). Expelling frogs and binding babies: Conception, gestation, and birth in nineteenth-century African-American midwifery. *World Archaeology, 45*(2), 272–284.

Women of valor: Emma Goldman—Women's rights—Birth control.
(n.d.). *Jewish Women's Archive.* Retrieved from https://jwa.org/
womenofvalor/goldman/womens-rights/birth-control

Chapter 3

Allen, R., & Cwiak, C. (2018). Contraception for women with medical
conditions. In: R. A. Hatcher, A. L. Nelson, J. Trussell, C. Cwiak,
P. Cason, M. S. Policar, . . . D. Kowal (Eds.), *Contraceptive technology*
(21st ed., pp. 543–560). New York, NY: Ayer.

American College of Obstetricians and Gynecologists. (2012). Risk
of venous thromboembolism among users of drospirenone-
containing oral contraceptive pills. Retrieved from https://
www.acog.org/Clinical-Guidance-and-Publications/
Committee-Opinions/Committee-on-Gynecologic-Practice/
Risk-of-Venous-Thromboembolism?IsMobileSet=false

American College of Obstetricians and Gynecologists. (2014). Depot
medroxyprogesterone acetate and bone effects. Retrieved from
https://www.acog.org/Clinical-Guidance-and-Publications/
Committee-Opinions/Committee-on-Adolescent-Health-Care/
Depot-Medroxyprogesterone-Acetate-and-Bone-Effects

American College of Obstetricians and Gynecologists. (2017, December
7). Practice advisory: Hormonal contraception and risk of breast
cancer. Retrieved from https://www.acog.org/Clinical-Guidance-
and-Publications/Practice-Advisories/Practice-Advisory-
Hormonal-Contraception-and-Risk-of-Breast-Cancer

Becker, B. J., & Betstadt, S. J. (2013). *Patient perception of safety of hormonal
contraception compared to pregnancy.* Paper presented at the 61st
annual clinical meeting of the American College of Obstetricians
and Gynecologists. New Orleans, LA.

Black, A., & Nelson, A.L. (2018). Contraception in the later reproductive
years. In R. A. Hatcher, A. L. Nelson, J. Trussell, C. Cwiak, P. Cason,
M. S. Policar, . . . D. Kowal (Eds.), *Contraceptive technology* (21st ed.,
pp. 561–578). New York, NY: Ayer.

Cortessis, V. K., Barrett, M., Brown Wade, N., Enebish, T., Perrigo, J.L.,
Tobin, J., . . . McKean-Cowdin, R. (2017). Intrauterine device use
and cervical cancer risk: A systematic review and meta-analysis.
Obstetrics & Gynecology, 130, 1226–1236.

Coutinho, E. M., & Segal, S. J. (1999). *Is menstruation obsolete?.*
New York, NY: Oxford University Press

Cwiak, C., & Edelman, A.B. (2018). Combined oral contraceptives (COCs). In R. A. Hatcher, A. L. Nelson, J. Trussell, C. Cwiak, P. Cason, M. S. Policar, . . . D. Kowal (Eds.), *Contraceptive technology* (21st ed., pp. 263–316). New York, NY: Ayer.

Davis-Floyd, R. (2003). *Birth as an American rite of passage.* Berkeley, CA: University of California Press.

Edelman, A., Micks, E., Gallo, M. F., Jensen, J. T., & Grimes, D. A. (2014). Continuous or extended cycle vs. cyclic use of combined hormonal contraceptives for contraception. *Cochrane Database of Systematic Reviews, 7.* doi:10.1002/14651858.CD004695.pub3

Faculty of Sexual and Reproductive Healthcare, Clinical Effectiveness Unit. (2019). Combined hormonal contraception. Retrieved from https://www.fsrh.org/standards-and-guidance/documents/combined-hormonal-contraception/

Gladwell, M. (2000, March 13). John Rock's error. *The New Yorker,* p. 52.

Hannaford, P. C., Iverson, L., Macfarlane, T. V., Elliot, A. M., Angus, V., & Lee, A. J. (2010). Mortality among contraceptive pill users: Cohort evidence from Royal College of General Practitioners' oral contraception study. *British Medical Journal, 340*(7748), c927. doi:10.1136/bmj.c927

Haraway, D. J. (2004). *The Haraway reader.* New York, NY: Routledge.

Hatcher, R. A., Nelson, A. L., Trussell, J., Cwiak, C., Cason, P., Policar, M. S., . . . Kowal, D. (Eds.). (2018). *Contraceptive technology* (21st ed.) New York, NY: Ayer.

Hillard, P. (2014). Menstrual suppression: Current perspectives. *International Journal of Women's Health, 6,* 631–637. doi:10.2147/IJWH.S46680

Horányi, D., Babay, L. E., Rigó, J., Jr., Győrffy, B., & Nagy, G. R. (2017). Effect of extended oral contraception use on the prevalence of fetal trisomy 21 in women aged at least 35 years. *International Journal of Gynecology & Obstetrics, 138,* 261–266.

Iversen, L., Sivasubramaniam, S., Lee, A. J., Fielding, S., & Hannaford, P. C. (2017). Lifetime cancer risk and combined oral contraceptives. *American Journal of Obstetrics and Gynecology, 216*(6), 580.e1–580.e9

Johnson, C. K. (2017, December 7). Birth control pills have been linked to an increased risk of breast cancer in new study. *The Independent.* Retrieved from: https://www.independent.co.uk/life-style/health-and-families/health-news/

breast-cancer-risk-birth-control-pills-oral-contraception-oestrogen-
levels-novo-nordisk-foundation-a8096661.html

Kaunitz, A. M., Pinkerton, J. V., & Manson, J. E. (2018). Hormonal
contraception and risk of breast cancer: A closer look. *Menopause,
25*, 477–479.

Lakehomer, H., Kaplan, P. F., Wozniak, D. G., & Minson, C. T. (2013).
Characteristics of scheduled bleeding manipulation with combined
hormonal contraception in university students. *Contraception, 88*(3),
426–430.

MacDorman, M. F., Mathews, T. J., & Declercq, E. (2012). Home births
in the United States 1990–2009. *NCHS Data Brief, 84*, 1–8.

Mansour, D., Gemzell-Danielsson, K., Inki, P., & Jensen, J. T. (2011).
Fertility after discontinuation of contraception: A comprehensive
review of the literature. *Contraception, 84*(5), 465–477.

Martin, E. (2001). *The woman in the body: A cultural analysis of
reproduction*. Boston, MA: Beacon Press.

Mørch, L. S., Skovlund, C. W., Hannaford, P. C., Iversen, L., Fielding,
S., & Lidegaard, Ø. (2017). Contemporary hormonal contraception
and the risk of breast cancer. *New England Journal of Medicine, 377*,
2228–2239.

Nagy, G. R., Gyrffy, B., Nagy, B., & Rigó, J., Jr. (2013). Lower risk for
Down syndrome associated with longer oral contraceptive use: A
case-control study of women of advanced maternal age presenting
for prenatal diagnosis. *Contraception, 87*(4), 455–458.

Nelson, A., & Shulman, L. Menstrual cycle: Normal patterns, menstrual
disorders, and menstrually-related problems. In R. A. Hatcher, A. L.
Nelson, J. Trussell, C. Cwiak, P. Cason, M. S. Policar, . . . D. Kowal
(Eds.), *Contraceptive technology* (21st ed., pp.1–62). New York,
NY: Ayer.

Picavet, C. (2014). Skipping the pill-free interval: Data from a Dutch
national sample. *Contraception, 89*(1), 28–30.

Pollock, D. (1999). *Telling bodies performing birth: Everyday narratives of
childbirth*. New York, NY: Columbia University Press.

Rabin, R. C. (2017, December 6). Birth control pills still linked to breast
cancer, study finds. *The New York Times.* Retrieved from: https://
www.nytimes.com/2017/12/06/health/birth-control-breast-
cancer-hormones.html

Rooks, J. (1999). *Midwifery and childbirth in America*. Philadelphia,
PA: Temple University Press.

Shah, H. (2018, October 16). A soaring maternal mortality rate: What does it mean for you? *Harvard Health Blog.* Retrieved from https://www.health.harvard.edu/blog/a-soaring-maternal-mortality-rate-what-does-it-mean-for-you-2018101614914

Solly, M. (2019, May 9). C.D.C says more than half of the U.S.' pregnancy-related deaths are preventable. *Smithsonian.com.* Retrieved from https://www.smithsonianmag.com/smart-news/cdc-says-more-half-us-pregnancy-related-deaths-are-preventable-180972140/

Strassmann, B. I. (1999). Menstrual cycling and breast cancer: An evolutionary perspective. *Journal of Women's Health, 8*(2), 193–202. doi:10.1089/jwh.1999.8.193

Study finds weak link between birth control and breast cancer. (2018, March). *Harvard Women's Health Watch.* Retrieved from https://www.health.harvard.edu/womens-health/study-finds-weak-link-between-birth-control-and-breast-cancer

Sundstrom, B. (2015). *Reproductive justice and women's voices: Health communication across the lifespan.* Lanham, MD: Lexington Books.

Thiel de Bocanegra, H., Chang, R., Menz, M., Howell, M., & Darney, P. (2013). Postpartum contraception in publicly-funded programs and inter-pregnancy intervals. *Obstetrics and Gynecology, 122,* 296–303.

U.S. Food and Drug Administration. (2012, April 10). FDA drug safety communication: Updated information about the risk of blood clots in women taking birth control pills containing drospirenone. Retrieved from https://www.fda.gov/drugs/drug-safety-and-availability/fda-drug-safety-communication-updated-information-about-risk-blood-clots-women-taking-birth-control

Vessey, M., Yeates, D., & Flynn, S. (2010). Factors affecting mortality in a large cohort study with special reference to oral contraceptive use. *Contraception, 82*(3), 221–229.

Wolf, J. H. (2011). *Deliver me from pain: Anesthesia and birth in America.* Baltimore, MD: Johns Hopkins University Press.

Zethraeus, N., Dreber, A., Ranehill, E., Blomberg, L., Labrie, F., von Schoultz, B., . . . Hirschberg, A. L. (2017). A first-choice combined oral contraceptive influences general well-being in healthy women: a double-blind, randomized, placebo-controlled trial. *Fertility and Sterility, 107*(5), 1238. doi:10.1016/j.fertnstert.2017.02.120

Chapter 4

American College of Obstetricians and Gynecologists. (2012). Over-the-counter access to oral contraceptives. ACOG Committee Opinion No. 544. American College of Obstetricians and Gynecologists. *Obstetrics & Gynecology, 120,* 1527–1531.

American College of Obstetricians and Gynecologists. (2015). Increasing access to contraceptive implants and intrauterine devices to reduce unintended pregnancy. ACOG Committee Opinion No. 642. American College of Obstetricians and Gynecologists. *Obstetrics & Gynecology, 126,* e44–e48.

American College of Obstetricians and Gynecologists. (2018a). Adolescents and long-acting reversible contraception: implants and intrauterine devices. ACOG Committee Opinion No. 735. American College of Obstetricians and Gynecologists. *Obstetrics & Gynecology, 131,* e130–e139.

American College of Obstetricians and Gynecologists. (2018b). The utility of and indications for routine pelvic examination. ACOG Committee Opinion No. 754. American College of Obstetricians and Gynecologists. *Obstetrics & Gynecology, 132,* e174–e180.

Birch, J. (2019, March 12). Why IUD insertions are so incredibly painful. *HuffPost.* Retrieved from: https://www.huffpost.com/entry/iud-insertion-pain_l_5c7fe889e4b0e62f69e8b919

Cauterucci, C. (2015, Nov. 30). "Pain on a cosmic level:" Getting an IUD can be excruciating. Is there a better way? *Slate.* Retrieved from: https://slate.com/human-interest/2015/11/getting-an-iud-can-be-insanely-painful-is-there-a-better-way.html

Cortessis, V. K., Barrett, M., Brown Wade, N., Enebish, T., Perrigo, J. L., Tobin, J., Zhong, C., . . . McKean-Cowdin, R. (2017). Intrauterine device use and cervical cancer risk: A systematic review and meta-analysis. *Obstetrics & Gynecology, 130,* 1226–1236.

Daniels, K. & Abma, J.C. (2018). Current contraceptive status among women aged 15–49: United States, 2015–2017. *NCHS Data Brief, 327.* Retrieved from https://www.cdc.gov/nchs/data/databriefs/db327-h.pdf

Epps, S. (Dir.). (2001). The one where Rachel tells . . . [TV episode]. *Friends.* Burbank, CA: Warner Bros. Studios.

Foster, D. G., Hulett, D., Bradsberry, M., Darney, P., & Policar, M. (2011). Number of oral contraceptive pill packages dispensed and subsequent unintended pregnancies. *Obstetrics & Gynecology, 117,* 566–572.

Gilliam M.L., Neustadt A., Kozloski M., Mistretta S., Tilmon S., & Godfrey E. (2010). Adherence and acceptability of the contraceptive ring compared with the pill among students: a randomized controlled trial. *Obstetrics & Gynecology, 115*, 503–510.

Guttmacher Institute. (2018). Contraceptive use in the United States [Fact sheet]. Retrieved from www.guttmacher.org.

McNicholas, C., Tessa, M., Secura, G., & Peipert, J.F. (2014). The contraceptive CHOICE project round up: What we did and what we learned. *Clinical Obstetrics & Gynecology, 57*(4), 635–643.

Mestad, R., Secura, G., Allsworth, J. E., Madden, T., Zhao, Q., & Peipert, J. F. (2011). Acceptance of long-acting reversible contraceptive methods by adolescent participants in the Contraceptive CHOICE Project. *Contraception, 84*, 493–498.

Qaseem, A., Humphrey, L. L., Harris, R. Starkey, M., & Denberg, T. D. (2014). Screening pelvic examination in adult women: A clinical practice guideline from the American College of Physicians. *Annals of Internal Medicine, 161*, 67–72.

Raifman, S., Barar, R., & Foster, D. (2018). Effect of knowledge of self-removability of intrauterine contraceptives on uptake, continuation, and satisfaction. *Women's Health Issues, 28*(1), 68–74.

Rosenstock, J. R., Peipert, J. F., Madden, T., Zhao, Q., & Secura, G. M. (2012) Continuation of reversible contraception in teenagers and young women. *Obstetrics & Gynecology, 120*, 1298–1305.

Secura, G. M., Allsworth, J. E., Madden, T., Mullersman, J. L., & Peipert, J. F. (2010). The contraceptive CHOICE project: Reducing barriers to long–acting reversible contraception. *American Journal of Obstetrics & Gynecology, 203*(115), e7.

Secura, G. M., Madden, T., McNicholas, C., Mullersman, J., Buckel, C. M., Zhao, Q., & Peipert, J. F. (2014). Provision of no-cost, long-acting contraception and teenage pregnancy. *New England Journal of Medicine, 371*, 1316–1323.

Stern, L. F., Simons, H. R., Kohn, J. E., Debevec, E. J., Morfesis, J. M., & Patel, A. A. (2015). Differences in contraceptive use between family planning providers and the U.S. population: Results of a nationwide survey. *Contraception, 91*(6), 464–469.

Sundstrom, B. (2012). Fifty years on "the pill": A qualitative analysis of nondaily contraceptive options. *Contraception, 86*(1), 4–11.

Sundstrom, B. (2015). *Reproductive justice and women's voices: Health communication across the lifespan.* Lanham, MD: Lexington Books.

Sundstrom, B., Baker-Whitcomb, A., & DeMaria, A. L. (2015). A qualitative analysis of long-acting reversible contraception. *Maternal and Child Health Journal, 19*(7), 1507–1514.

Sundstrom, B., Billings, D., & Zenger, K.E. (2016). Keep calm and LARC on: A theory-based long-acting reversible contraception (LARC) access campaign. *Journal of Communication in Healthcare, 9*(1), 49–59.

Tyler, C. P., Whiteman, M. K., Zapata, L. B., Curtis, K. M., Hillis, S. D., & Marchbanks, P. A. (2012). Health care provider attitudes and practices related to intrauterine devices for nulliparous women. *Obstetrics & Gynecology, 119,* 762–771.

Chapter 5

Addams, Jane. (1912). A New Conscience and an Ancient Evil. New York: The Macmillan Company. Accessed at Project Gutenberg, https://www.gutenberg.org/files/15221/15221-h/15221-h.htm.

Aiken, A. R. A., & Scott, J. (2016). Family planning policy in the United States: The converging politics of abortion and contraception. *Contraception, 93*(5), 412–420. doi:10.1016/j.contraception.2016.01.007

American College of Obstetricians and Gynecologists. (n.d.). Birth control (contraception): Resource overview. Retrieved from https://www.acog.org/Womens-Health/Birth-Control-Contraception

American College of Obstetricians and Gynecologists. (2013, November). Health care for homeless women. Retrieved from https://www.acog.org/Clinical-Guidance-and-Publications/Committee-Opinions/Committee-on-Health-Care-for-Underserved-Women/Health-Care-for-Homeless-Women?IsMobileSet=false

American Public Health Association. (n.d.). About APHA. Retrieved from https://www.apha.org/about-apha

American Public Health Association. (2015, November 3). Universal access to contraception. Retrieved August 15, 2019, from https://www.apha.org/policies-and-advocacy/public-health-policy-statements/policy-database/2015/12/17/09/14/universal-access-to-contraception

Arons, J. (2012, February 21). The high costs of birth control: A major barrier to access. *Rewire.News.* Retrieved from https://rewire.news/article/2012/02/21/high-costs-birth-control/

Ashbee, E. (2014). *The Bush administration, sex and the moral agenda.* Oxford, England: Manchester University Press.

Barber, J. S., Ela, E., Gatny, H., Kusunoki, Y., Fakih, S., Batra, P., & Farris, K. (2019). Contraceptive desert? Black_White differences in characteristics of nearby pharmacies. *Journal of Racial and Ethnic Health Disparities, 6*(4), 719–732. doi:10.1007/s40615-019-00570-3Barot, S. (2015, November 17). Moving oral contraceptives to over-the-counter status: Policy versus politics. *Guttmacher Policy Review, 18*(4). Retrieved from https://www.guttmacher.org/gpr/2015/11/moving-oral-contraceptives-over-counter-status-policy-versus-politics

Barrett, J. B., Da Vanzo, J., Ellison, C. G., & Grammich, C. (2014). Religion and attitudes toward family planning issues among US adults. *Review of Religious Research, 56*(2), 161–188.

Beaton, C. (2017, April 18). Why does America have fewer types of IUDs than other countries? *The Atlantic.* Retrieved from https://www.theatlantic.com/health/archive/2017/04/why-america-has-fewer-iuds-than-other-countries/523077/

Bell, J. (2019, January 2). Why trans men, nonbinary, and genderqueer people use birth control. *Clue.* Retrieved from https://helloclue.com/articles/cycle-a-z/why-trans-non-binary-and-genderqueer-people-use-birth-control

Block, J. (2017, July 26). Some call this contraceptive a breakthrough for women: Others say it's dangerous. *Washington Post.* Retrieved from http://www.washingtonpost.com/sf/style/2017/07/26/essure/

Center for Global Health. (n.d.). What types of organizations are working in Global Health? Retrieved from https://www.albany.edu/globalhealth/working-in-global-health-orgs.php

Conley, J. (2019, August 19). Trump's domestic gag rule forces Planned Parenthood to withdraw from Title X funding, threatening healthcare of 1.5 million women. *Common Dreams.* Retrieved from https://www.commondreams.org/news/2019/08/19/trumps-domestic-gag-rule-forces-planned-parenthood-withdraw-title-x-funding

Corey, E. K., Frazin, S., Heywood, S., & Haider, S. (2017). Homeless women's desire for and barriers to obtaining effective contraception. *Contraception, 96*(4), 287. doi:10.1016/j.contraception.2017.07.095

Critchlow, D. T. (1999). *Intended consequences: Birth control, abortion, and the federal government in modern America.* New York, NY: Oxford University Press.

Deckman, M., & McTague, J. (2015). Did the "war on women" work? Women, men, and the birth control mandate in the 2012 presidential election. *American Politics Research, 43*(1), 3–26. doi:10.1177/1532673X14535240

Dockterman, E. (2014, July 1). Supreme Court Hobby Lobby contraception ruling: What women should know. *Time.* Retrieved from https://time.com/2941323/supreme-court-contraception-ruling-hobby-lobby/

Does your Medicare plan include birth control coverage? (n.d.). *Medicare.org.* Retrieved from https://www.medicare.org/articles/does-your-medicare-plan-include-birth-control-coverage/

Driver, A. (2018, November 13). See the migrant caravan arriving in Mexico City. *Time.* Retrieved from https://time.com/longform/migrant-caravan-mexico/

Fleury, A. (2016, May 4). Fleeing to Mexico for safety: The perilous journey for migrant women. *United Nations University.* Retrieved from https://unu.edu/publications/articles/fleeing-to-mexico-for-safety-the-perilous-journey-for-migrant-women.html

Grindlay, K. (2016, November 6). A guide to birth control when you're in the military. *Bedsider.* Retrieved from https://www.bedsider.org/features/967-a-guide-to-birth-control-when-you-re-in-the-military

Guttmacher Institute. (2016, March 14). Insurance coverage of contraceptives. Retrieved from https://www.guttmacher.org/state-policy/explore/insurance-coverage-contraceptives

Hagerty, B. B. (2009, March 29). In Quiverfull movement, birth control is shunned [Audio file]. *PBS: Morning Edition.* Retrieved from https://www.npr.org/templates/story/story.php?storyId=102005062

Indian Health Services. (n.d.). About IHS. Retrieved from https://www.ihs.gov/aboutihs/

Indian Health Services. (2015, October 15). Emergency contraception. In *Indian health manual* (Chapter 15). Retrieved from https://www.ihs.gov/IHM/pc/part-1/p1c15/

Kaiser Family Foundation. (2015, July 10). Private and public coverage of contraceptive services and supplies in the United States. Retrieved from https://www.kff.org/womens-health-policy/fact-sheet/private-and-public-coverage-of-contraceptive-services-and-supplies-in-the-united-states/

Kaiser Family Foundation. (2019a, May 3). Poll finds most Americans oppose the Trump administration's changes to restrict Title X family planning funds from clinics that also provide or refer for abortion. Retrieved from https://www.kff.org/womens-health-policy/press-release/poll-finds-most-americans-oppose-trump-administrations-changes-to-restrict-title-x-family-planning-funds-from-clinics-that-provide-or-refer-for-abortion/

Kaiser Family Foundation. (2019b, July). The U.S. government and international family planning and reproductive health efforts. Retrieved from https://www.kff.org/global-health-policy/fact-sheet/the-u-s-government-and-international-family-planning-reproductive-health-efforts/

Lieber, C. (2018, August 14). The first "birth control app" was just approved by the FDA. Its transparency and effectiveness are in question. *Vox.* Retrieved from https://www.vox.com/2018/8/14/17684392/natural-cycles-birth-control-app-fda

Lipton-Lubet, S. (2014). Contraceptive coverage under the Affordable Care Act: Dueling narratives and their policy implications. *American University Journal of Gender, Social Policy & the Law,* 22(2), 343–385.

McCammon, S. (2019, August 19). Planned Parenthood withdraws from Title X program over Trump abortion rule [Audio file]. *NPR: All Things Considered.* Retrieved from https://www.npr.org/2019/08/19/752438119/planned-parenthood-out-of-title-x-over-trump-rule

Men's health and the Affordable Care Act: What's covered? (2018, November 1). *Bedsider.* Retrieved from https://www.bedsider.org/features/862-men-s-health-and-the-affordable-care-act-what-s-covered

Newport, F. (2012, May 22). Americans, including Catholics, say birth control is morally OK. *Gallup.* Retrieved from https://news.gallup.com/poll/154799/Americans-Including-Catholics-Say-Birth-Control-Morally.aspx

Office of Women's Health. (2014, April 17). Making birth control better, safer, and more accessible for women. In *30 achievements in women's health in 30 years (1984–2014).* Retrieved from https://www.womenshealth.gov/30-achievements/16

Oregon Health Authority. (n.d.). Reproductive Health Equity Act: Reproductive and sexual health. Retrieved from https://www.oregon.gov/oha/PH/HEALTHYPEOPLEFAMILIES/REPRODUCTIVESEXUALHEALTH/Pages/reproductive-health-equity-act.aspx

Paul VI. (1968, July 25). *Humanae vitae*. Retrieved from http://
w2.vatican.va/content/paul-vi/en/encyclicals/documents/hf_p-
vi_enc_25071968_humanae-vitae.html

Pear, R., Ruiz, R. R., & Goodstein, L. (2017, October 6). Trump
administration rolls back birth control mandate. *The New York
Times*. Retrieved from https://www.nytimes.com/2017/10/06/us/
politics/trump-contraception-birth-control.html

Pharmacists refusing to fill spark national controversy. (2015,
August 12). *Pharmacy Times*. Retrieved from https://www.
pharmacytimes.com/contributor/alex-barker-pharmd/2015/08/
pharmacists-refusing-to-fill-spark-national-controversy

Planned Parenthood. (n.d.). [Homepage]. Retrieved from https://www.
plannedparenthood.org

Powell, N. (2017, October 31). 3 reasons why we need to talk about
queer and trans people and birth control. *Everyday Feminism*.
Retrieved from https://everydayfeminism.com/2017/10/
queer-trans-birth-control/

Power to Decide. (n.d.). Access to birth control. Retrieved from https://
powertodecide.org/what-we-do/access/access-birth-control

Richman, A. R., Daley, E. M., Baldwin, J., Kromrey, J., O'Rourke,
K., & Perrin, K. (2012). The role of pharmacists and
emergency contraception: Are pharmacists' perceptions
of emergency contraception predictive of their dispensing
practices? *Contraception, 86*(4), 370–375. doi:10.1016/
j.contraception.2012.01.014

Rugg, J., & Barry, D. (2015, February 4). Access to contraception
for women serving in the armed forces. *Center for American
Progress*. Retrieved from https://www.americanprogress.
org/issues/women/reports/2015/02/04/106121/
access-to-contraception-for-women-serving-in-the-armed-forces/

Silliman, J., Fried, M. G., Ross, L., & Gutiérrez, E. (2016). *Undivided
rights: Women of color organizing for reproductive justice*. Chicago,
IL: Haymarket Books.

Snyder, A. H., Weisman, C. S., Liu, G., Leslie, D., & Chuang, C. H.
(2018). The impact of the Affordable Care Act on contraceptive use
and costs among privately insured women. *Women's Health Issues,
28*(3), 219–223. doi:10.1016/j.whi.2018.01.005

Solinger, R. (2013). *Reproductive politics: What everyone needs to know*.
New York, NY: Oxford University Press.

United Nations Family Planning Association. (n.d.). About us. Retrieved from https://www.unfpa.org/

U.S. Department of Veterans Affairs. (n.d.). Women veterans health care: Long-acting reversible contraceptives. Retrieved from https://www.womenshealth.va.gov/WOMENSHEALTH/OutreachMaterials/ReproductiveHealth/Contraception.asp

Washington, J. (2019, August 12). "I couldn't afford anything": Title X transformed this woman's life, but it may not be an option for much longer. *Mother Jones*. Retrieved from https://www.motherjones.com/politics/2019/08/title-x-emma-bosley-planned-parenthood-donald-trump-gag-rule/

Weldon, K. (2014, July 7). Public attitudes about birth control. Updated December 6, 2017. *HuffPost*. Retrieved from https://www.huffpost.com/entry/public-attitudes-about-bi_b_7880080

Women Refugee Commission. (n.d.). Family planning. Retrieved from https://www.womensrefugeecommission.org/srh-2016/family-planning/

World Health Association. (2018, February 8). Family planning/contraception. Retrieved from https://www.who.int/news-room/fact-sheets/detail/family-planning-contraception

World Health Organization. (2013). *Family Planning, 351*. Retrieved from http://www.who.int/mediacentre/factsheets/fs351/en/

Wyer, M., Barbercheck, M., Cookmeyer, D., Ozturk, H., & Wayne, M. (Eds.). (2014). *Women, science, and technology: A reader in feminist science studies*. New York, NY: Routledge.

Zimmerman, J. (2015). *Too hot to handle: A global history of sex education*. Princeton, NJ: Princeton University Press.

Conclusion

Alley Team. (n.d.). Femtech companies innovating women's healthcare. *Alley*. Retrieved August 29, 2019, from https://www.alley.com/post/meet-the-femtech-companies-innovating-traditional-womens-health

American College of Obstetricians and Gynecologists. (2019). Over-the-counter access to oral contraceptives. *Obstetrics & Gynecology, 134*(4), 886–887.

Center for Connected Health Policy. (n.d.). About telehealth. Retrieved from https://www.cchpca.org/about/about-telehealth

Curtis, K. M., Tepper, N. K., Jamieson, D. J., & Marchbanks, P. A. (2013). Commentary: Adaptation of the World Health Organization's selected practice recommendations for contraceptive use for the United States. *Contraception, 87,* 513–516. doi:10.1016/j.contraception.2012.08.024

Dutta, M. J. (2007). Communicating about culture and health: Theorizing culture-centered and cultural sensitivity approaches. *Communication Theory, 17*(3), 304–328. doi:10.1111/j.1468-2885.2007.00297.x

Dutta, M. J. (2015). Decolonizing communication for social change: A culture-centered approach. *Communication Theory, 25*(2), 123–143. doi:10.1111/comt.12067

Free the Pill. (n.d.). [Homepage]. Retrieved from http://freethepill.org/

Gava, G., & Meriggiola, M. C. (2019). Update on male hormonal contraception. *Therapeutic Advances in Endocrinology and Metabolism, 10.* doi:10.1177/2042018819834846

Grossman, D. (2015). Over-the-counter access to oral contraceptives. *Obstetrics and Gynecology Clinics of North America, 42*(4), 619–629. doi:10.1016/j.ogc.2015.07.002

Guttmacher Institute. (2015, November 17). Moving oral contraceptives to over-the-counter status: Policy versus politics. Retrieved from https://www.guttmacher.org/gpr/2015/11/moving-oral-contraceptives-over-counter-status-policy-versus-politics

Health Resources and Services Administration, Maternal and Child Health. (2017, April 1). (SDAR) Disability-related disparities in sex education, contraceptive use and unintended pregnancy. Retrieved from https://mchb.hrsa.gov/research/project_info.asp?ID=306

Kaunitz, A. M. (2008). Hormonal contraception in women of older reproductive age. *New England Journal of Medicine, 358*(12), 1262–1270. doi:10.1056/NEJMcp0708481

Light, A., Wang, L.-F., & Gomez-Lobo, V. (2017). The family planning needs of young transgender men. *Journal of Pediatric and Adolescent Gynecology, 30*(2), 274. doi:10.1016/j.jpag.2017.03.012

Karsten, J., & West, D. (2018, September 12). Telehealth apps expand access for reproductive health care. Brookings Institution. Retrieved from https://www.brookings.edu/blog/techtank/2018/09/12/telehealth-apps-expand-access-for-reproductive-health-care/

Male birth control pill passes human safety tests. (2019, March 25). *Drug Discovery From Technology Networks.* Retrieved from https://www.technologynetworks.com/drug-discovery/news/male-birth-control-pill-passes-human-safety-tests-317223

Mendez, I. M., Averett, P. E., & Lee, J. G. L. (2018). Messaging lesbian, gay, bisexual, and transgender health inequities: A qualitative exploration: *Health Promotion Practice, 20*(1), 18–21. doi:10.1177/1524839918809009

mHealthIntelligence. (2018, February 8). Mobile health program helps Chicago reach underserved adolescents. Retrieved from https://mhealthintelligence.com/news/mobile-health-program-helps-chicago-reach-underserved-adolescents

OCs OTC Working Group. (n.d.). FAQs. Retrieved from http://ocsotc.org/faqs/

Parekh, J., Finocharo, J., Kim, L., & Manlove, J. (2019). Pregnancy prevention program for males. *Education Digest, 84*(8), 48–54.

Sundstrom, B., DeMaria, A. L., Ferrara, M., Meier, S., & Billings, D. (2019). "The closer, the better:" The role of telehealth in increasing contraceptive access among women in rural South Carolina. *Maternal and Child Health Journal, 23*(9), 1196–1205. doi:10.1007/s10995-019-02750-3

Sundstrom, B., Smith, E., Vyge, K., Miletich, A., Benigni, G., & Delay, C. (2018, Nov.). Formative audience research to understand women's perspectives of providing oral contraceptives (OCs) over-the-counter (OTC) in rural South Carolina. American Public Health Association (APHA) Annual Meeting; Sexual and Reproductive Health (SRH) Section, San Diego, CA.

What is telehealth? (2018, February 1). *NEJM Catalyst*. Retrieved from https://catalyst.nejm.org/what-is-telehealth/

INDEX